Teeth for Life for Older Adults

Quintessentials of Dental Practice – 7
Prosthodontics - 1

Teeth for Life for Older Adults

By
P Finbarr Allen

Editor-in-Chief: Nairn H F Wilson
Editor Prosthodontics: P Finbarr Allen

Quintessence Publishing Co. Ltd.

London, Berlin, Chicago, Copenhagen, Paris, Milan, Barcelona,
Istanbul, São Paulo, Tokyo, New Dehli, Moscow, Prague, Warsaw

British Library Cataloguing in Publication Data

Allen, P. Finbarr
  Teeth for life for older adults. - (The quintessentials of dental practice)
  1. Aged - Dental care 2. Prosthodontics
  I. Title II. Wilson, Nairn H. F.
  618.9'776

ISBN 1850970564

ISBN 1-85097-056-4

Foreword

With many more people living longer, remaining dentate – albeit, partially dentate – throughout life and having ever-increasing oral-health expecta- tions, the dental care of the mature adult patient is one of the major chal- lenges of present-day general dental practice. *Teeth for Life for Older Adults* – Volume 7 of the Quintessentials for General Dental Practitioners Series – gets to the heart of this challenge: effective management of the older patient, long-term treatment planning, countering the effects of oral ageing, the maintenance of typically heavily restored and often worn dentitions, and dealing with the many, varied prosthodontic dilemmas the mature adult patient may pose.

A very large and immensely important subject area in contemporary dentistry is succinctly captured in this attractive book. As in all the volumes in the Quin- tessentials for General Dental Practitioners Series, the easy-to-read text is gen- erously illustrated with high-quality informative images. The care of mature adult patients is often difficult and may be fraught with problems. This book recognises the great diversity of clinical issues that may arise in the provision of this care and provides sound guidance on how best to achieve favourable clinical outcomes in the management of patients in the older age groups. A further hallmark of the books in the Quintessentials for General Dental Prac- titioners Series is an emphasis on information that may find immediate chair- side application. *Teeth for Life for Older Adults* is no exception in this regard, as it is packed full of answers to the multitude of questions practitioners ask about the management of mature adult patients. *Teeth for Life for Older Adults* is a most welcome and important addition to the dental literature.

Nairn Wilson
Editor-in-Chief

Preface

As the population ages, dentists will have to provide care for larger numbers of older adults. Improvements in dental health have led to increasing numbers of dentate older adults, but there is a high burden of maintenance associated with ageing dentitions. Older adult patients will present a range of challenges and demands. There will be fewer new edentulous patients, but the threat of total tooth loss will remain a reality for significant numbers of adults for the foreseeable future. Dentists will be expected to provide care for these patients in an era of diminishing resources for healthcare. This text, using currently available clinical and research-based evidence, aims to give the general dental practitioner an insight into the management of older adults. The first chapter gives an overview of the problems experienced by the edentulous patient. The presentation, aetiology and diagnosis of common disease states affecting the dentate older adult are then discussed and management strategies are outlined. The final chapter covers the use of complete overdentures and invites the reader to consider whether this should be the end-point of dental treatment for older adults.

Having Read This Book

It is hoped that having read this book the reader will be able to:
- Understand the consequences of total tooth loss and the desirability of avoiding edentulousness if at all possible.
- Recognise that there is an expanding older adult population who are retaining more of their teeth than ever before, and that much of this older population are not willing to accept tooth loss as an inevitable consequence of ageing.
- Recognise that there are many threats to the goal of healthy ageing of the oral tissues.
- Recognise that health promotion as well as disease prevention is an important aspect of clinical care in this population.
- Understand that ill health is not an inevitable part of ageing and that complex treatment is not contraindicated in older adults.
- Understand that long-term treatment planning is essential to avoid total tooth loss at an advanced age.

- Recognise that, for some older adults, it is acceptable to limit treatment goals to provide a functional rather than a complete dentition.
- Recognise the importance of thinking strategically if edentulousness is to be avoided. If roots are to be retained to support an overdenture, this should be the final phase in long term treatment planning.

P Finbarr Allen

Acknowledgements

I would like to thank the following people for their help in the preparation of this book: Dr Frank Burke, Dr John Whitworth and Mr Mike Milward for contributing chapters; Professor Iain Chapple for his help in the preparation of Chapter 4, Dr Edith Allen for proof reading the entire text; Dr Nick Jepson, Mr David Murray and Mr Francis Nohl for permission to use some of their photographs as illustrations in the text. Finally, I want to acknowledge my former colleagues at the University of Newcastle upon Tyne, UK for inspiring my interest in gerodontology.

Contents

Chapter 1
The Edentulous State

Aim

Population studies indicate that the proportion of dentate older adults is increasing dramatically in industrialised countries. This chapter aims to provide a view of changing patterns of oral health of older adults in industrialised countries.

Outcome

At the end of this chapter, the practitioner should be aware of the consequences of edentulism and the desirability of avoiding total tooth loss in older adults.

What is an "Older Adult"?

It is often said that age is a state of mind, and to a degree there is no consensus as to what constitutes an "older adult". Some authors have classed adults over the age of 60 as young elderly (60–75 years old) and older elderly (> 75 years old). In this book, an older adult is arbitrarily over the age of 65 years. It should, however, be remembered that planning to maintain teeth for life in older adults starts much sooner than this. In the past, a large proportion of adults had lost all of their teeth long before this age. Improving adult oral health has led to increasing numbers of adults retaining teeth later in life, but oral disease levels in this age group remain high. Consequently, dentists need to plan early and strategically to face the many challenges posed to maintaining teeth for life in older adults.

Epidemiology

The percentage of the population over the age of 65 years is increasing in countries in the industrialised world. This is a reflection of increased life expectancy and the approach of middle age for the "baby boom" generation. In the United Kingdom, for example, the mean age of the population is expected to rise from 38.4 years in 1996 to nearly 42 years by 2021. The number of adults over the age of 65 years is projected to increase by 2.7 million during the same time frame. The proportion of the "elderly" elderly (i.e. aged 85 years and over) in the UK is also expected to rise, from approximately 800,000 in 1991 to 1.5 million in the year 2010.

The dental status of older adults is also changing dramatically. In 1968, 37% of adults (aged 16 years and over) in England and Wales were edentulous. By 1988, this figure for the whole of the UK was 21% and figures from the 1998 UK Adult Dental Health survey show that 13% of the adult population are edentulous. Long-term predictions indicate that the prevalence of edentulousness in the UK will eventually level out at 6% by the year 2028.

The level of edentulousness at the present time is strongly associated with dental problems of the distant past, with those who were rendered edentulous 30 to 40 years ago strongly influencing the edentulous statistic. As the population is generally ageing, and as it takes a long time for age cohorts to pass through the population, it will be some time before edentulousness will be a thing of the past. An examination of the most recent UK Adult Dental Health survey in 1998 shows that one-fifth of the 55–64 age cohort were edentulous, with this fraction rising to three-fifths of the over-75-year-old adults. Even if dental clearances stopped now, which is unlikely, it would take until 2038 before edentulousness was eradicated. While the proportion of the dentate adult UK population has increased, the DMFT index score for cohorts over the age of 45 has not substantially changed. In terms of periodontal health, 75% of the 35–44-year-old cohort had periodontal pocketing, 13% of which were classified deep pockets. These data suggest that the burden of maintenance of heavily restored dentitions will remain a major requirement for the dental profession.

A further factor to consider is the attendance pattern of adults, and their attitudes to dental care. At the present time, significant proportions of adults do not attend the dentist regularly, and only attend when in pain or when they need emergency treatment. Barriers to the uptake of dental care include cost, fear of dental procedures and negative images of the dental practice environment. It seems likely that many in this group of adults will remain a "hard core" of non-attenders, and are unlikely to remain dentate throughout their lifetime.

Attitudes to Edentulousness

The attitude to tooth loss is also changing. Greater numbers of adults are reporting that they find the thought of losing their teeth upsetting and are

2

likely to seek treatment to retain some of their natural teeth. Owing to the high prevalence of dental disease in the older-age cohorts, many will not achieve their aim of being dentate for life. Consequently, the loss of natural teeth will, for some, occur late in life at a time when denture control skills are difficult to acquire.

The attitudes to edentulousness, and satisfaction with complete dentures will, in the future, be influenced by current trends in adult dental health. As the proportion of adults retaining teeth into old age increases, the transition to the edentulous state will, for some, occur later in life. As the ability to learn the complex series of reflexes required to control complete dentures diminishes with age, it seems possible that denture-wearing complaints may increase in the elderly age groups.

Anatomical Consequences of Edentulousness

The anatomical changes which occur following extraction of natural teeth can broadly be divided into intraoral and extraoral changes. These will differ between individuals who remain partially dentate and those who are edentulous following tooth loss. As people age, loss of alveolar bone is inevitable. However, following total tooth loss, alveolar bone resorption is greatly increased. Alveolar bone height and width decrease markedly (Figs. 1-1 and 1-2). Most of this change occurs in the first year following extractions, but remains an inexorable process throughout life. Resorption occurs on the buccal aspect of the maxillary ridge and the lingual aspect of the mandibular ridge. In a mixed longitudinal study over 25 years, Tallgren demonstrated the extent of bone loss in edentulous individuals. She demonstrated that the loss of bone is four times greater in the mandible than the maxilla. Despite

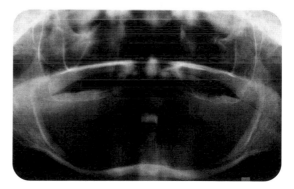

Fig 1-1 Orthopantomogram showing the edentulous jaws of a 62-year-old female. Note how thin the lower jaw is following extensive loss of alveolar bone.

3

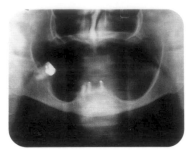

Fig 1- 2 Orthopantomogram of 75-year-old female with retained dental roots in the anterior mandible. Note the bone height around teeth compared to edentate areas in the lower jaw.

extensive research, the reason for great individual variation in bone loss remains unclear. It seems likely that a combination of local and systemic factors may be responsible for this phenomenon.

As well as anatomical changes, further consequences of tooth loss include:
- impaired mastication
- limitation of food selection, especially nutritious foods such as fruit and vegetables
- speech impairment
- appearance change
- psychosocial impact.

The influence of tooth loss on *masticatory ability*, performance and dietary selection has been well documented. Objective tests of *masticatory performance* indicate that chewing efficiency of edentulous adults is approximately 20% that of a dentate individual.

Subjective tests that assess patients' attitudes to food choice suggest that edentulous patients tend to favour highly flavoured soft foods that are of low nutritional value. Reasons for this are complex, and include socio-economic factors as well as denture-related causes. Surveys of nutritional intake, report that edentulous adults have lower intake of fibre, vitamin C and other important nutrients, compared with dentate adults. This suggests that edentulous patients with poor-quality diet are at a higher risk of serious illness, including cardiovascular disease and cancer.

Loss of anterior teeth affects *speech* and can be a difficult problem to deal with, particularly in patients with a skeletal Class 2 jaw relationship.

In addition to preserving bone, teeth support soft tissues such as the cheeks and lips. This in turn has an influence on *appearance*, and appearance is adversely affected once teeth are lost. This is most noticeable in the circumoral region, as the commisures of the lips collapse inward. A further consequence is loss of vertical dimension and this has the affect of approximating the nose to the chin (Fig 1-3). Complete replacement dentures can rectify some of these changes, but there are limitations. In cases of severe resorption, it may be impossible to meet the patient's aesthetic requirements and at the same time provide stable replacement dentures.

Increasingly, researchers are beginning to look at wider issues of health-related *quality of life*. As well as impacting on function, it is now recognised that tooth loss has much broader social and psychological impacts. Acceptance of tooth loss and complete replacement dentures is variable and subjective. In the area of oral health, this research indicates that patients who have lost their natural teeth have poorer oral health-related quality of life than patients with their own teeth. From a clinical point of view, the outcome of complete removable dentures in the rehabilitation of edentulousness is difficult to predict. As just described, there are a number of difficult functional problems to rectify, and yet some patients manage very well with technically inadequate dentures. It would appear that satisfaction with the outcome is not strongly correlated with the technical quality of dentures or the denture-bearing tissues. Some studies also indicate that patients with

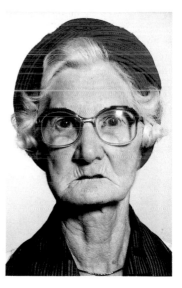

Fig 1-3 Appearance of edentulous patient. Note loss of vertical dimension and resultant proximity of chin to nose.

5

denture-wearing difficulties score highly on neuroticism indices. Whilst complete replacement dentures continue to be successful for many patients, there are significant numbers of edentulous patients for whom complete replacement dentures will not be satisfactory.

Alternatives to Complete Replacement Dentures: Implant-retained Prostheses

The use of osseointegrated dental implants has greatly improved the management of edentulous patients. Prostheses retained on dental implants allow the possibility of overcoming some of the limitations of complete replacement dentures. However, before assuming that implant-retained prostheses are the natural end-point for treatment, there are a number of factors which the clinician should consider, namely:

- How does the patient feel about surgery? Many older patients are anxious about surgery and may refuse treatment.
- Is the patient prepared to pay the costs involved in implant therapy?
- Does the patient have sufficient bone to place implants? Bone grafting may be required and this could be a barrier to treatment.
- If bone grafting is required, this prolongs treatment time. Is the patient prepared to accept this?
- Is the patient prepared to accept the burden of maintenance associated with implant-retained prostheses?

Implant-retained prostheses are an important and significant advance in the management of tooth loss. However, it should not be assumed that they are desirable or accessible for all older adults, and attempts should be made to retain a natural, health-functioning dentition for life. A further issue that the clinician may have to resolve is when there has been evidence of chronic periodontal disease. In this situation, gradual bone loss occurs and this may increase complexity of implant therapy at a later date. The timing of how and when tooth loss occurs could be critical, and should be carefully considered. Monitoring the signs of progression of periodontal disease is vital, and if response to therapy is poor, and maintenance of tissue health is not possible, then tooth loss may have to be planned sooner rather than later.

Future Directions

Maintaining a healthy, functional dentition for life is one of the goals for oral health of the World Health Organization, and this should be a major aim of all dental and oral health care professionals. Satisfactory oral health is not simply dependent on removing pathology, and a minimum number of teeth are required to maintain functional and psychosocial well-being. Current research suggests that 20 teeth with between three and five occluding pairs of posterior teeth is the minimum requirement for older adults. Part of the dentist's role in maintaining overall health is to ensure that adults retain as much of their dentition in a healthy state as long as is practicable. This means that dentists need to plan care for the long as well as short term, thinking strategically how such an aim can be achieved.

Conclusions

- Increasing numbers of adults are retaining teeth into old age.
- Many adults have dentitions requiring a high degree of maintenance.
- Edentulousness is decreasing, but there will be a need to provide complete dentures for some time to come.
- Loss of all natural teeth has functional and psychosocial consequences and may impact significantly on health-related quality of life.
- Patient acceptance of complete replacement dentures is difficult to predict and dependent on many varied factors.
- Dentists will need to think strategically in their efforts to maintain teeth for life in older adults.
- Implant-retained prostheses may be of benefit, but could also be beyond the financial resources of older adults. Older adults may also be reluctant to have surgery to place implants and to accept the burden of maintenance of implant-retained prostheses in old age.

Further Reading

Kelly M, Steele JG, Nuttall N. et al. Adult Dental Health Survey UK 1998. London. Office of National Statistics, 2000.

Zarb GA, Bolender C, Carlsson GE. Prosthodontic Treatment for Edentulous Patients. 11th ed. St Louis: Mosby, 1997.

Chapter 2
Changing Times: The Dentate Elderly

Aim

The aim of this chapter is to describe current trends in the dental status of the elderly, including factors influencing attitudes to oral healthcare in this age group.

Outcome

At the end of this chapter, the practitioner should be aware that tooth retention in older adults is increasing. In addition, oral health of older adults is variable and presents a range of clinical challenges. It seems likely that edentulousness will be less acceptable to current and future older adults than in the past. The practitioner will have to determine the level of oral function that is acceptable to individual patients and plan care accordingly. It should be recognised that some older adults will still lose their teeth, and in this situation a controlled progression to edentulism should be planned.

Attitudes to Teeth: Influences on Patients

It seems likely that the current generation of older adults has greater expectations of oral health than previous generations. In the past, the vast majority of older adults were edentulous and a significant portion of dentists' time was spent rehabilitating edentulous older adults. Recent adult dental health surveys indicate that older adults no longer consider total tooth loss as an inevitable consequence of old age, and increasing numbers of older adults are likely to be distressed at the thought of losing all of their natural teeth. They are less likely to accept complete removable dentures, and will be better informed about treatment options. The clinician may be asked to provide complex restorations and should not be inhibited from doing so if it is considered an appropriate treatment option. It is important to remember that old age is not inevitably associated with ill health and that advancing years is not necessarily a contraindication to treatment such as implant-retained restorations. Trends indicate that total tooth loss tends to cluster in socio-economically deprived areas. In more affluent areas, older adults are more likely to seek restorative dental treatment to maintain compatibility with their peers. A further influence on older adults is the opinion of their family. The clinician may find that they have to explain treatment options to immediate family members, as they have an influence on the patient's ability to attend for treatment and may also be the financial provider for the patient.

The clinician should also be conscious of the apparent divergence of opinion between demands of older adults and professionally assessed treatment need. This phenomenon has been described in many parts of the medical and dental literature, and suggests that acceptance of advice and treatment from health care professionals is not unquestioned.

Dentate Older Adults: Are They All the Same?

The range of treatment options available for older adults depending on dental status is shown in Fig 2-1.

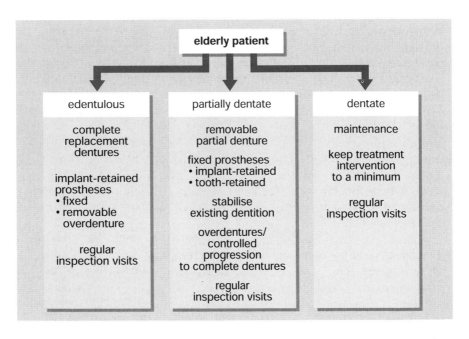

Fig 2-1 Possible treatment options for the older adult depending on dental status.

10

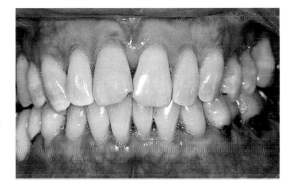

Fig 2-2 Healthy dentition of a 74-year-old, dentally aware female patient. Low maintenance is required.

The elderly dentate population can present in a variety of dental states. These can be characterised as follows.

The dentally-aware, low-maintenance patient

The dentally aware, low-maintenance patient will have been fairly resistant to dental disease. They may have lost some periodontal support, but generally have very little periodontal pocketing. A number of teeth may have been heavily restored or have full coverage crown restorations. Very few, if any, teeth have been extracted and those that have been lost may be replaced by fixed bridgework. These patients are usually very dentally aware, and practise satisfactory plaque-control measures. Such a patient is seen in Fig 2-2. This is a 74-year-old lady who has attended regularly for dental inspection visits. Her periodontal state is excellent, and her oral hygiene impeccable. She has had some conventional and resin-bonded bridgework to replace missing teeth in her lower jaw. She requested replacement of these missing teeth as she felt her chewing ability and appearance were affected by losing teeth. Otherwise, her dental health was excellent. Such a patient requires routine inspections once or twice a year, and should have very few problems with her teeth.

The dentally-aware, high-maintenance patient

Other patients may be dentally aware, but have been more susceptible to dental disease and thus require more maintenance. They may have already lost a significant number of teeth, and had these replaced with removable partial dentures (RPDs) or extensive fixed bridgework retained on teeth or implants. There may have been significant loss of periodontal attachment and some teeth may show signs of mobility. The history given by the patient may indicate that tooth loss has been gradual or possibly that they have had a stable dentition for a long period of time. The patient shown in Fig 2-3 is

11

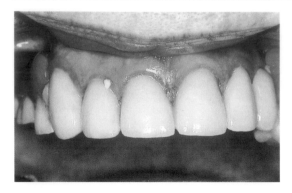

Fig 2-3 Dentition of an elderly patient who is dentally aware but requires high maintenance. Her maxillary posterior teeth have been replaced with a precision attachment retained removable partial denture and she has anterior porcelain-fused-to metal crowns.

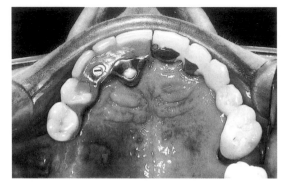

Fig 2-4 Extensive treatment involving implants. This elderly patient was anxious to avoid removable dentures. (Courtesy of Mr F Nohl)

an example of such a case. This 65-year-old lady has extensive porcelain-fused-to-metal crownwork on her maxillary anterior teeth. The distal units have extracoronal precision attachments to retain an RPD. These are the second generation of restorations, and she has had the current restorations for approximately two years. This patient has satisfactory appearance and oral function, but requires regular maintenance. The vitality of heavily restored teeth, particular those restored with crowns, will also have to be monitored. She will be a high consumer of dental care for the remainder of her life but, if she can maintain satisfactory oral hygiene, she should retain her surviving natural dentition.

With the increasing availability of dental implants, some older patients will have teeth replaced by implant-retained restorations. The patient shown in Fig 2-4 had fixed bridgework on both sides of the maxillary arch. One of the retainer teeth on the left of her maxilla fractured, and the bridge had to be removed. An attempt to replace missing teeth with an RPD proved unsuccessful, and an implant-retained bridge was provided. Patients such as this will require maintenance of components as well as soft tissues around the transmucosal elements of the implant restorations. Current research indicates that these restorations have a good long-term prognosis, and old age does not necessarily influence implant therapy outcomes. In a partially dentate patient, the periodontal support of the natural dentition will require maintenance.

The clinician should be aware that oral health status in older adults might be adversely affected by changes in medical status. Conditions that affect the patient's ability to remove plaque or alter flow of saliva are a particular threat. These consequences are discussed in more detail in Chapter 3.

The dentally unaware patient

The final group of older partially dentate adults include those who visit dentists on an irregular basis. These patients can be divided into two broad categories:

* patients who only attend the dentist when in pain
* patients who are not concerned about their teeth.

The distinction between these groups of patients may have significance for the type of treatment the clinician may provide. In the first category, the main disincentive to dental treatment could be fear of dental procedures. A further problem could be the financial cost of treatment. These patients will avoid visiting the dentist and only attend for emergency treatment. In many cases, they are unhappy with their dental status, and may be unable to perform normal functions of daily living such as speaking and eating to their satisfaction. Despite this, they will usually request the simplest and most expedient form of treatment possible. The perceived barrier to care is compounded by poor communication between dentist and patient. If time were spent discussing the problems of the patient in a less intimidating environment than the dental surgery, these patients may be more amenable to having comprehensive dental care. For many older adults, the experience of sitting in a dental chair can be intimidating, and this may not be the most appropriate place to discuss dental treatment options.

The irregular attenders in the second category are usually unconcerned about their teeth. They may have lost many of their teeth, or show signs of advanced dental disease. Plaque control may be very poor, and total tooth loss may be inevitable. Some of these patients may be relatively resistant to dental diseases and, despite poor oral hygiene, may not have experienced loss of periodontal support or extensive dental caries. There may be signs of advanced pathological tooth wear, and a number of teeth may have over-erupted or drifted into tooth spaces. Although their appearance may be significantly compromised by tooth loss or pathological tooth wear, these patients may be relatively unconcerned about their dental state. In a number of cases, the patient may only seek a dentist's opinion to satisfy a spouse or other close relative. These patients are usually not well motivated, and will not be interested in complex dental treatment. If they agree to treatment, then it may be difficult to plan how to replace missing teeth. Problems that the clinician may face include:

- lack of space for restorations
- lack of neutral zone into which denture teeth can be placed
- unstable occlusion
- poor-quality denture-bearing tissues.

The unknown factor in trying to assess these patients is how much dental treatment they will tolerate. For example, in Fig 2-5, the patient had been an irregular attender for many years. However, he had had teeth extracted in an ill-considered fashion, and gradually lost all antagonistic occluding contacts. This eventually started to cause stripping of his palatal mucosa and pain and food impaction finally influenced the patient to seek more comprehensive treatment. From the clinical point of view, the occlusion was completely unstable, and the anterior teeth have been weakened by tooth wear and are heavily restored. The patient requested the simplest treatment possible. As will be discussed in a later chapter, long-term treatment planning would have avoided this consequence of dental extraction and made the outlook less doubtful.

These patients are likely to be low consumers of dental care. If they can be sufficiently motivated, more comprehensive treatment could be considered

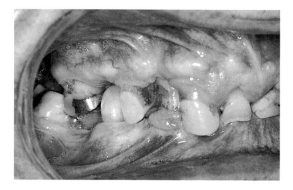

Fig 2-5 Deranged occlusion of a patient who attended irregularly for dental treatment. Note the loss of all antagonistic occlusal contacts.

14

at a later date. In the early stages, priority should be given to providing a stable dentition that is relatively easy to maintain. The situation can then be re-evaluated and, if appropriate, a further course of treatment may be considered.

Controlled Transition to the Edentulous State

If the response to initial therapy and patient compliance has been poor, then there may be no alternative but to plan progression to complete replacement dentures *in a controlled fashion*. Gradual progression to edentulousness increases the chances of successful adaptation to wearing complete dentures. As the patient is unlikely to accept a period of healing without replacement of teeth, immediate replacement dentures will be required. The goal of immediate denture therapy is to maintain satisfactory appearance and function during the post-extraction phase of treatment. The clinical and laboratory stages of providing complete immediate replacement dentures involve:

- Discussion of the consequences of tooth loss with the patient and explaining clearly the treatment plan. The patient must understand that the tissues will change during the healing period following dental extractions and that frequent adjustment of the dentures may be required. The patient must also be advised that immediate dentures are intended to be temporary, and will probably have to be replaced after six to twelve months
- Provision of transitional RPDs to replace mainly posterior teeth in the first instance. These should be designed carefully to ensure they are as retentive and stable as possible (Fig 2-6).
- After a suitable transitional period (six months is usually sufficient), the clinician may convert the transitional partial dentures to complete immediate replacement dentures. An impression should be recorded with the dentures in situ. Measure the periodontal pockets to give the dental

Fig 2-6 Transitional partial denture. Note the use of clasps to increase retention and comfort of the prosthesis.

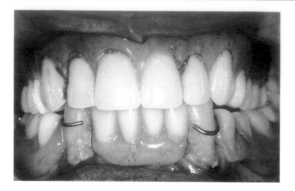

Fig 2-7 Insertion of complete immediate replacement denture following extraction of remaining natural maxillary teeth.

technician an indication of the anticipated tissue collapse following extraction of the teeth. If a complete immediate replacement is made de novo, then an impression should be made of the remaining natural teeth and tissues in a customised tray. Jaw registration and trial denture stages are also required.

- In the dental laboratory, the technician prepares the cast by removing the anterior teeth and scribing the cast using the periodontal pocket depth measures as a guide. Teeth are waxed onto the cast and partial dentures, flasked, packed and processed.
- The finished complete dentures are returned to the clinic. The clinician extracts the remaining natural teeth and inserts the complete immediate dentures (Fig 2-7). Normal post-extraction instructions are provided.
- The patient is instructed to leave the dentures in situ for the next 24 hours. An appointment is arranged for the following day to inspect the dentures, the tissues and make minor adjustments.
- The patient is advised to take the dentures out only for cleaning and to continue full-time wear for a further week.
- At one-week review, further adjustments to occlusion and peripheral extensions may be required.
- Review at one month. Adjust as necessary, bearing in mind that the denture should not traumatise the tissues. A chairside reline using a resilient or hard liner may be required at this stage or during the next six months.
- After six months, a definitive treatment plan is made. At this stage the usual treatment option would be to provide new replacement dentures. Occasionally, it is possible to rebase the immediate replacement dentures.

Conclusions

- Tooth loss is not an inevitable consequence of old age.
- Dental health of the elderly is variable, and a number of treatment strategies may be used to maintain satisfactory oral function.
- Total tooth loss may be inevitable in some older adults. Transition to the edentulous state should be planned in a controlled fashion.
- Implant-retained prostheses can be provided for the older adult. Some older adults may refuse implant therapy on the grounds of financial cost or fear of surgery.

Chapter 3
Threats to Oral Health in Older Adults

Aim

The aim of this chapter is to outline potential threats to the ideal of retaining teeth for life. A further aim of this chapter is to describe how dentists and auxiliary staff can promote oral health in the older adult.

Outcome

The practitioner should be aware of the need to plan care for life, not just the short term. They should recognise that a number of conditions increase in prevalence in old age and threaten tooth survival. By planning care with this in mind, it is possible to maintain a natural, functioning dentition for life. At the end of this chapter, the practitioner should understand pathological conditions affecting the soft tissues that can occur in the older patient and how these may be prevented with vigilance and timely advice. The importance of health promotion by the dental team should also be recognised.

Factors Leading to Increased Tooth Retention by Older Adults

The improvement in tooth retention rate as reported in surveys of adult dental health could be attributed to a number of factors. These include:
- improved awareness of oral health
- improved access to dental care
- oral health promotion by the dental profession
- fluoridation of toothpastes
- fluoridation from local (e.g. mouth rinses) and systemic (fluoridation of water supplies) sources.

The influence of fluoride on adult oral health is particularly dramatic in young and middle-aged adults and, as these cohorts age, tooth retention is likely to increase further.

Threats to Oral Health

There are many potential threats to oral health in older adults, and these are summarised in Fig 3-1.

Tooth retention

Whilst improvement is welcome, there are a number of significant threats to oral health in older adults. Many adults have teeth that have been heavily restored, and the burden of maintaining heavily restored dentitions will remain significant for many years. This factor, coupled with the tendency for older adults to find plaque control more difficult to maintain with age, poses a significant threat to the dentition of older adults. A further consideration is the reticence of older adults to attend a dentist on a regular basis, and this will require thought from policymakers in the future. In the past, older adults tended to accept deterioration of their teeth as an inevitable consequence of ageing. However, promotion of healthy ageing is now made more straightforward using mass communication media including the internet. Health promotion may also be facilitated by members of the dental team designated to undertake this process as part of the patient's overall care. Finally, the importance of prevention cannot be overemphasised.

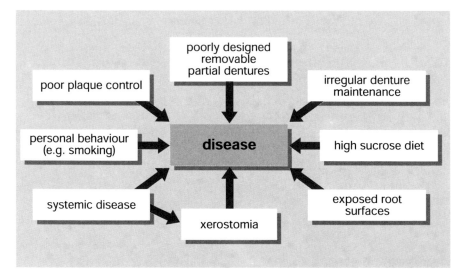

Fig. 3-1 Factors that threaten oral health in older adults.

Common clinical problems in older adults that pose a threat to retention of teeth are:

- Periodontal disease
- Root caries
- Tooth wear
- Poorly designed removable prostheses
- Systemic diseases.

Plaque control tends to diminish with age, mainly due to loss of manual dexterity. *Periodontal disease* is not an inevitable consequence of ageing, but the effects of cumulative periodontal attachment loss may become apparent in old age in patients susceptible to periodontal disease. Periodontal disease and the elderly will be described in greater detail in Chapter 4.

The prevalence of *root caries* is increasing as more adults retain teeth into old age. This is partly explained by the increased tooth retention by older adults and partly due to other environmental factors. Recession of the gingival tissues exposes the root-surface dentine and predisposes the patient to caries. This risk increases with the presence of RPDs, age and reduced salivary flow. The aetiology, diagnosis and treatment of root caries will be discussed in greater detail in Chapter 5.

Pathological (as opposed to normal physiological) *tooth wear* is a threat to the vitality of teeth. The prevalence of tooth wear in adults has increased, and this may be explained mostly by lifestyle and dietary changes that have taken place over the past 20 to 30 years. Management strategies for tooth wear in older adults are considered in more detail in Chapter 6.

RPDs that have been well designed, constructed and maintained pose minimal threat to oral health. However, many studies show that RPDs are associated with high levels of caries and periodontal disease. Plaque levels increase markedly in the presence of RPDs and, in the absence of meticulous plaque-control measures, oral disease can be the consequence. A particular problem is the tissue-supported acrylic denture commonly known as the "gum stripper". This tissue-supported prosthesis (Fig 3-2) has been prescribed widely, mainly due to its low cost and ease of repair. A significant problem arises when these dentures are not maintained or regularly reviewed. As the underlying alveolar ridge resorbs, the denture sinks into the tissues. This in turn "strips" the gingival tissues, leading to exposure of the underlying root surfaces (Fig 3-3). Consequently, these types of prosthesis, especially in the lower jaw, can hasten the process of tooth loss.

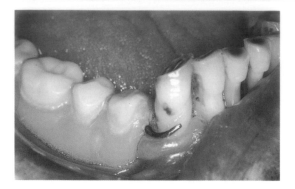

Fig 3-2 Tissue-supported, free-end saddle removable partial denture. Note the sinking of the denture into the tissues. (Courtesy of Mr ID Murray)

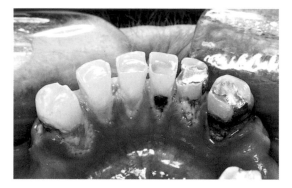

Fig 3-3 Damage caused by poorly maintained tissue-supported free-end saddle removable partial denture. Note the inflamed gingival margins, exposure and carious lesions on root surfaces. (Courtesy of Mr ID Murray)

Tooth-supported dentures can also affect oral health. A common fault is to encroach upon the gingival tissues with components of the denture such as connectors and clasp tips (Fig 3-4). This in turn causes plaque accumulation and predisposes the patient to caries and gingival inflammation. However, when partial dentures are carefully designed, and plaque control is adequate, research indicates that it is possible to maintain good oral health in the presence of RPDs. When providing RPDs, prevention of disease can be aided by:

- Providing tooth support for the denture where possible. In cobalt-chromium-based dentures, rests should be placed on the tooth surfaces adjacent to the saddles. Wrought rests can be incorporated into acrylic-based RPDs to provide tooth support.
- Minimising coverage of the dental and gingival tissues. Essentially, keep the design of the RPD as simple as possible. The connector should not encroach on the gingival margins of the teeth, and clasps should not cover

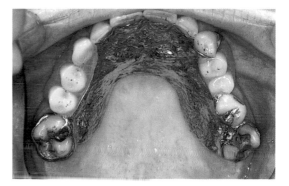

Fig 3-4 Extensive coverage of the denture-bearing tissues with the major connector of the denture. This is likely to damage the tissues, particularly the gingival margins.

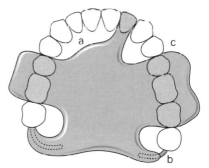

Fig 3-5 Design features of Every style acrylic removable partial denture. The key features of this design are: (a) relief of the connector from the standing teeth; (b) wrought clasps engaging the distal surface of the last standing teeth; (c) good proximal contact with natural teeth.

exposed root surfaces. Every design of acrylic dentures can be provided in the maxilla (Fig3-5).

- Carefully instructing the patient in cleaning techniques for both RPD and the natural teeth. This includes careful instruction in oral-hygiene procedures, encouraging the patient to clean the denture after meals and to use denture cleaners.
- Arranging regular inspection visits and checking the fit of the RPD to ensure that it is not causing damage. The frequency of these inspection visits depends on the individual patient, but at least one inspection visit per year is recommended.

A number of *systemic diseases* impact on the oral health of older adults. These can affect the intraoral environment or cause extraoral changes (e.g. arthritis of the hands) that make oral hygiene procedures difficult. Patients with arthritic conditions (Fig 3-6) affecting the hands often require specially modified toothbrushes to facilitate plaque removal. Some medications cause

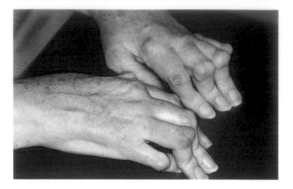

Fig 3-6 Patient with rheumatoid arthritis affecting her fingers. This patient struggles to use a conventional toothbrush and requires a modified toothbrush to clean her teeth.

xerostomia (dry mouth) and thus the buffering capacity of saliva is dramatically altered. Examples of medications commonly prescribed for the elderly that may cause dry mouth are shown in Table 3-1. Whilst this table is not exhaustive, it can be seen that dry mouth is a common side-effect of these medications, and the reader is referred to the British National Formulary for a more comprehensive listing of drugs with oral side-effects.

Caries and periodontal disease increase when saliva flow decreases, and teeth tend to wear at a greater rate. Depending on the severity of xerostomia, the

Table 3-1 Commonly prescribed drugs that may cause xerostomia (dry mouth).

Drug	Generic name	Conditions
beta blockers	propanolol	hypertension
ACE inhibitors	lisinopril	hypertension
diuretics	frusemide	hypertension; chronic heart failure
calcium channel blockers	nifedipine	hypertension; stable angina
hypnotics	diazepam	anxiety
antidepressants	amitryptiline	depression
anti-Parkinson's	carbidopa	Parkinson's disease

tongue may appear lobulated or fissured, and the buccal mucosa may appear dry (Fig 3-7). Further difficulties caused by xerostomia are an increase in discomfort with RPDs, burning mouth sensation, taste changes and problems chewing, speaking and swallowing. Soft-tissue pathology is also a potential consequence, and *candidal infection* is often seen in patients with dry mouth. In some cases, it may be possible to liaise with a patient's general medical practitioner to change their medication to one less likely to cause xerostomia or perhaps to alter the dose of the medication and so decrease the severity of the unwanted side-effect.

Occasionally, xerostomia is one of the symptoms associated with diseases such as Sjogren's Syndrome or degenerative salivary gland disorders, or as a consequence of irradiation of a tumour in the head and neck region. This should be confirmed by recording a thorough medical history and, if an underlying condition has yet to be diagnosed, the dentist should liaise with the patient's medical practitioner. For both clinician and patient, management of xerostomia can be particularly difficult, and palliative treatment is all that can be achieved. Possible strategies for dealing with the effects of xerostomia are:

- stimulation of saliva flow with citric acid or lemon juice
- use of high viscosity saliva substitutes, e.g. Saliva Orthana, Oral Balance
- use of paraffin wax or chewing gums
- use of cholinergic agents such as pilocarpine
- reservoir dentures.

None of these remedies is ideal, and a process of trial and error may be required to select the most effective regime for the patient. In some cases,

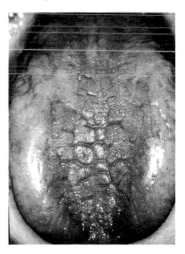

Fig 3-7 Lobulation and fissuring of tongue seen in a patient with xerostomia. (Courtesy of Mr ID Murray)

advising the patient to use frequent sips of water is sufficient. Unwanted side-effects may be associated with use of acidic agents (erosive tooth wear) or chewing gums containing sorbitol (diarrhoea). Acidic agents should not be recommended for dentate patients, and saliva substitutes may be more appropriate. It is unclear how effective salivary substitutes are in relieving the symptoms of dry mouth, and some research indicates that they may not be effective. They have the advantage of being easy to carry in a pocket or handbag and can be sprayed onto the oral mucosa as required. The use of cholinergic agents such as pilocarpine must only be considered following consultation with the patient's physician. These have some side-effects, such as sweating and polyuria. Finally, in edentulous patients with xerostomia, a reservoir can be incorporated into one of the complete dentures. A saliva substitute can be placed into the reservoir that then leaks into the oral cavity during the course of the day. This has been shown to be of some benefit, but will slightly increase the bulk of the denture.

An essential part of any strategy to deal with xerostomia is to try to prevent dental disease. In addition to instruction in plaque-removal techniques, these patients should be encouraged to try to keep the mouth moist throughout the day by taking frequent sips of water. Daily fluoride mouth rinses (0.05% sodium fluoride) should also be recommended and they may require regular professional application of fluoride gels in a customised acrylic tray, depending on the severity of caries and the frequency of new lesions.

Oral Pathology

Oral cancer
Oral cancer is a relatively uncommon condition, but appears to be increasing in prevalence, particularly in older adults. It is associated with significant morbidity and a poor survival rate if not detected early. The sites most commonly affected by cancer are the lips followed by the tongue. Tumours affecting the tongue and floor of mouth metastasise quickly and are associated with a low survival rate. Depending on the stage of the disease, survival at 5 years can be as low as 50%, making it one the most lethal of tumours. Approximately 90% of oral carcinomas are squamous cell carcinoma. It is vital that the dental practitioner carefully checks the oral tissues at each inspection visit for any signs of neoplasia or premalignant changes such as leukoplakia or erythroplakia. Ulceration, with a raised, rolled edge, and induration around the periphery of the lesion, are characteristic features of oral cancer (Fig 3-8). Lesions are occasionally exophytic and leukoplakic lesions may also be adjacent to the tumour. Lesions can be related to the periphery of a denture (Fig

3-9), and this should be suspected if the lesion does not resolve following relief of the denture.

If an ulcer with this appearance is detected, the clinician should question the patient about the history of the ulcer. Malignant ulcers are frequently painless and the symptom duration reported is not as one would expect given the size of the lesion. Cervical lymph nodes should also be carefully examined and enlarged, hard and fixed lymph nodes should be regarded as very suspicious. If the lesion has been present for more than one week, the patient should be referred for specialist opinion. Once a diagnosis of carcinoma has been made, treatment usually involves wide surgical excision in combination with radiotherapy. Chemotherapy is sometimes used in the management of oral carcinoma.

The general dental practitioner has a major role to play in the management of these patients before and after the treatment of the tumour. Radiother-

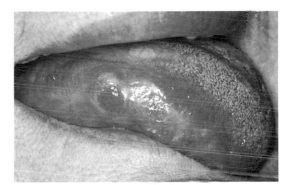

Fig 3-8 Squamous cell carcinoma affecting the lateral surface of the tongue. (Courtesy of Mr ID Murray)

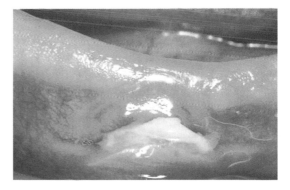

Fig 3-9 Squamous cell carcinoma associated with the periphery of a mandibular complete replacement denture. (Courtesy of Mr ID Murray)

apy has a number of unpleasant side-effects in the oral cavity, as many of the minor salivary glands may be damaged by the treatment. This causes:
- mucositis
- xerostomia (dry mouth)
- trismus of the jaw muscles
- radiation induced caries can occur if the reduction of salivary flow is severe.

The following advice and management strategy should be employed by the general dental practitioner in treating a patient prior to and during a course of radiotherapy:

- Prior to radiotherapy, the dentist should ensure that all dental disease is treated. Teeth with a poor prognosis should be extracted prior to radiotherapy, as extraction following radiotherapy in the region of the oral cavity is undesirable. The blood supply to jaw bone may be compromised by radiotherapy, and osteoradionecrosis may be a consequence of a dental extraction during or shortly after radiotherapy.
- A vigorous programme of maintenance is required post-radiotherapy to prevent the need for dental extractions. If extractions are required, specialist surgical advice should be obtained. Teeth should be extracted as atraumatically as possible under antibiotic prophylaxis.
- Application of fluoride gels (e.g. 0.4% stannous fluoride gel) in a vacuum-formed tray will help prevent radiation-induced caries. Daily use of fluoride mouth rinses (e.g. Colgate Fluorigard™) to prevent dental caries should be encouraged and oral hygiene instruction should also be given.
- Chlorhexidine mouth rinses should be recommended to help with plaque control, but may be contraindicated if mucositis is evident.
- Mucositis is a painful condition, and treated symptomatically with anaesthetic mouth rinses (e.g. benzydamine hydrochloride), as required. Careful brushing of the teeth with a soft brush should be recommended and Water-Pik irrigators may also be of benefit.
- Topical antifungal lozenges (amphoteracin B) can also be of benefit in the management of mucositis. A soft diet should be recommended and the patient should avoid alcohol.
- Dietary advice, such as minimising sucrose intake, should be given to reduce the risk of caries.
- Treat carious lesions early.
- Prescribe jaw muscle exercises to reduce muscle trismus. The use of wooden tongue spatulas is helpful. The patient should put as many of these between the teeth as possible and gradually increase the number to increase jaw opening.

Oral cancer: the role of health promotion

Even with conservative management, surgical excision of an oral tumour can result in significant loss of oral function and quality of life. Without doubt, prevention is better than cure, and the dental team can play a pivotal role in promoting a healthy lifestyle. A major aetiological factor in the development of oral cancer is cigarette smoking, and combining smoking with regular alcohol consumption significantly enhances this. Members of the dental team can help reduce the prevalence of oral cancer by encouraging patients to cease smoking and reduce alcohol consumption. This may be done in conjunction with a general medical practitioner. As much support as possible should be offered to the patient in this endeavour.

Denture-induced Pathology

Research has shown that plaque levels increase in the presence of RPDs. The patient needs to have careful oral hygiene instruction, as previously described. Pathological conditions are also associated with continuous denture wear, particularly ill-fitting dentures. Instructions that should be given include:

- Remove and clean the denture and the teeth after meals.
- Remove the denture at night and soak in a denture cleaner.
- Use of fluoride mouth rinses in patients at moderate to high risk of developing dental caries.
- Hypochlorite-containing agents corrode metal-based dentures and should only be used with acrylic dentures.
- Do not soak dentures in boiling water as this causes bleaching of the acrylic.
- Do not scrub acrylic dentures with toothpaste or hard brushes, as this scratches the acrylic and can cause staining.

Denture cleaners can be categorised according to the principal cleaning agent (Table 3-2). There is some debate as to their effectiveness, and also concern regarding their effect on permanent and temporary soft lining materials. Hypochlorite solutions appear to cause least damage to soft lining materials, but may bleach acrylic resin and cause corrosion of metal bases. Alkaline peroxide cleaners are probably the most damaging to soft lining materials.

Candidal infection

Candidal infections of the oral cavity can be either chronic or acute. Chronic conditions are more common, are usually painless and have a multifactorial aetiology (Fig 3-10). They are defined by the denture-bearing area (Fig 3-11), which is a diagnostic feature, and only affect the maxillary jaw. Chronic

Table 3-2 Commonly used denture-cleaning agents.

Agent	Mechanism of action	Examples of brand names
alkaline peroxide	effervescence dislodges foreign material	Steradent™
acid cleaners	softens debris	Denclen™
hypochlorite cleaners	bleaching	Dentural™

candidal infection in the mouth is sometimes associated with angular chelitis (Fig 3-12). Other causes of angular chelitis are staphyloccal infection from the nasal cavity or iron-deficiency anaemia. Treatment of a chronic candidal infection includes:

- Denture-hygiene advice, including the use of one of the denture cleaners described in Table 3-2.
- Advising the patient not to wear their dentures at night when asleep. Patients should also be encouraged to clean their dentures with a soft brush and warm soapy water (not with toothpastes: see above).
- Reducing trauma to the tissues, which involves using conditioners on the fitting surface of the denture to improve adaptation to the tissues. The tissue conditioner should not be left longer than 3-4 weeks, as they will dete-

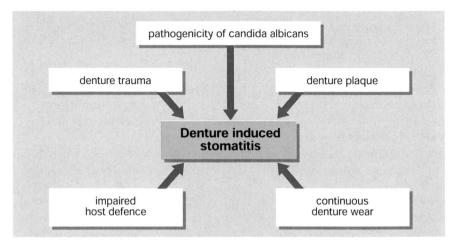

Fig 3-10 Aetiological factors in chronic candidal infection affecting the oral palatal mucosa.

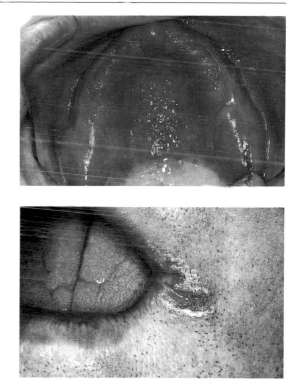

Fig 3-11 Chronic candidal infection defined by the denture-bearing area in an edentulous patient.

Fig 3-12 Angular chelitis affecting the corner of the mouth. This patient had a dry mouth and chronic candidal infection of the denture-bearing tissues.

riorate and cause further trauma to the tissues after this period of time.
- Using topical antifungal agents (e.g. miconazole) when fungal infection is confirmed. Systemic antifungal agents should not be prescribed without consulting the patient's physician.

In most cases, a new denture is indicated. Ideally, the denture-induced candidal infection should be fully resolved prior to recording of impressions.

Denture granuloma

This is also known as denture hyperplasia, and is caused by chronic irritation of the mucosa, usually by an overextended denture (Fig 3-13). The patient should be encouraged to leave the denture out of the mouth as much as possible, and the clinician should remove the area of overextension. Small lesions will usually resolve within two months. Large lesions may not resolve completely, and may have to be removed surgically. This should be undertaken with care, as surgical removal will lead to scar tissue and this may further compromise the retention of the denture. The clinician should also be

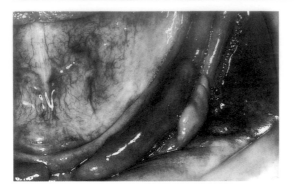

Fig 3-13 Area of denture-induced hyperplasia associated with an overextended denture periphery. (Courtesy of Mr ID Murray)

vigilant for potential neoplastic change in these lesions and consider sending a biopsy of the lesion for a pathology report if unsure of the diagnosis.

Timing of denture replacement

There is no consistency in the literature regarding the lifespan of removable dentures. This is not surprising as individual patient circumstances differ. However, it is important to emphasise the need for patients who wear dentures to attend for regular inspection appointments. This will enable the clinician to check for faults in the dentures, health of the teeth and periodontal tissues and also soft tissue pathology. Occasionally, the patient may have suffered a medical complaint that may compromise their oral health since their last visit. In this situation, the appropriate advice may be given to help prevent dental disease.

Health Promotion and Disease Prevention

The preceding chapters have highlighted the major changes that have occurred in the oral health of older adults in recent years. Tooth retention has increased substantially in an ageing population. Prevalence of root caries and periodontal diseases is increasing in older adults in an era of diminishing resources for health care. A further consideration is that many older adults will not end their lives living independently and will have to be looked after by carers. At the present time, oral health of older adults is not as good in persons living in institutions. Consequently, preventive strategies and health promotion will be required to reduce treatment need.

The general dental practitioner has an important role to play in providing domiciliary services for these patients, and visits by dental hygienists to institutions or old patients in their homes is also of benefit. A service such as this can be facilitated by the use of portable equipment including hand pieces. Resources for oral health care are diminishing and disease prevention has a vital role to play in ensuring satisfactory oral health care for all older adults. The strategy for achieving this should include:

- Long-term treatment planning.
- Thinking strategically to avoid total tooth loss in old age.
- Regular maintenance, including oral hygiene instruction and dietary advice.
- Involvement of the dental team, including dental hygienist, and use of patient information literature to promote oral health.
- Offering domiciliary visits to institutions and old people living at home.

Conclusions

- There is a significant burden of dental maintenance in older adults.
- There are a number of clinical disease states that threaten teeth in older adults. Preventive measures will be vitally important in protecting teeth against the consequences of dental and systemic disease.
- Health promotion has an important role to play in maintaining a healthy dentition for life. Older patients should be reviewed regularly to check for oral pathology.
- Vigilance essential, particularly in older patients who smoke as early detection of cancer is critical.

Chapter 4
Ageing and Periodontal Disease

Aims

This chapter aims to give the practitioner an insight into the issues involved in managing older patients with periodontal diseases. It covers:

- The frequency with which periodontal diseases are seen in the older population.
- The biological age changes that take place in the periodontium.
- The older patient's attitude to periodontal diseases.
- How these factors interrelate in the clinical management of periodontal disease in older patients.

Outcomes

Having read this chapter the practitioner should understand what age changes take place in the periodontal tissues, and how these relate to the management of such patients.

Introduction

As outlined in Chapter 1, increases in life expectancy, patient expectations, and the longevity of the natural dentition are likely to place increasing demands on practitioners for periodontal therapy. It is important to have a sound knowledge of the biology of ageing in relation to the periodontal tissues in order to achieve tooth retention for longer and thus facilitate more-effective restorative treatment plans. This chapter outlines the key biological effects on the periodontal tissues and summarises their impact on clinical management in practice.

How Big is the Problem?

With regard to periodontal disease the most recent adult dental health survey published in the UK (1998) reported that patients over 65 years showed the highest incidence of loss of attachment, with 38% of patients over the age of 65 experiencing attachment loss of over 5.5mm. This compares with an average incidence for all dentate subjects of 10%. It is, however, important to recognise that this loss of attachment is due to the cumulative effects of disease progression over a period of time, rather than being a consequence of the ageing process. (This is an important point, which will be discussed later in this chapter.)

The Range of Age Changes Seen in the Periodontium

Extensive research over a number of years has identified a number of changes that are commonly observed in the periodontium with increasing age. When discussing the periodontal tissues it should be remembered this includes the gingival tissues (epithelium and connective tissue), cementum, alveolar bone as well as the periodontal ligament. These tissues, and how ageing alters them, will now be discussed in more detail.

The Gingival Tissues

The gingival tissues comprise both epithelial and connective tissues.

Epithelium

A number of research groups have demonstrated that the epithelial tissues become thinner with age, and this is accompanied by a reduction in the degree of keratinisation of the epithelial tissue. A more controversial finding relates to the rate of turnover of the gingival epithelium. Research in this area has produced inconsistent findings, with some groups noting a reduction in turnover rate while others have found no change or even an increase in cell proliferation. Clinically, the gingivae do appear to become less stippled, but the clinical relevance of this is as yet uncertain.

Connective tissue

With regard to the underlying connective tissue of the gingivae, the main age-related features are a reduction in cellularity, along with a change in texture from a fine to a dense and coarser connective tissue. Researchers have also proposed that the rate of collagen synthesis reduces with increasing age.

These findings may affect how the gingivae respond to periodontal disease progression or indeed therapy, but to date there is no convincing evidence that these histological findings have any direct clinical implications.

Cementum

Cementum is laid down on the root surface throughout life and a number of studies have found that the thickness of cementum increases with age. This is true for the whole root surface but is found to be more pronounced in the apical third region, possibly as a response to passive eruption of the dentition.

The Periodontal Ligament

The periodontal ligament consists of cells, fibres and ground substance, all of which show histological age-related changes. Periodontal fibroblast proliferation, along with collagen and protein synthesis, is reduced, resulting in a less-cellular periodontal ligament. A number of research groups have noted a difference in the width of the periodontal ligament with an increase in age but this has subsequently been related to occlusal loading of teeth rather than being an age change *per se*.

Alveolar Bone

A number of changes have been demonstrated within alveolar bone. These include a reduction in cellularity, a reduction in the thickness of the cribiform plate, as well as the surface of the alveolar bone in contact with the periodontal ligament becoming "jagged", with a less regular insertion of collagen fibres.

Age-related Changes to Dental Plaque

Both quantitative and qualitative microbiological changes have been observed with increasing age. For example, the number of viable microorganisms reduces with age; the number of spirochetes increases, and a reduction in streptococci has also been reported. Other age-related changes in the structure and function of dental plaque have been observed:
- An increase in rate of plaque accumulation and formation.
- Increases in immunological factors (e.g. IgA, IgM, complement component C3, lysozyme) have been demonstrated in plaque harvested from older patients.

These factors are interesting but their importance in terms of susceptibility to, and the natural history of, periodontal disease has yet to be determined.

Immune Response Within the Periodontal Tissues

Another area of interest is the manner in which age impinges on the host's ability to respond to disease, and in this case, periodontal disease. Extensive research has been published examining how the immune system changes with age. In periodontal diseases this may have an impact on the host's response to a microbial challenge with periodontal pathogens, which may affect the natural history of the periodontal disease process. It has been proposed by several authors that the immune response is reduced in older patients, and this may result in an increase in susceptibility to a number of diseases including periodontal disease.

Healing Capacity of the Periodontium

There has been extensive literature published on healing responses and increasing age, with the majority of authors concluding that healing is compromised in older subjects. However, clinical studies of patients with periodontal disease seem to show that age is not a significant factor in healing and, in fact, the major determinant in such cases is the subject's inherent susceptibility to periodontal disease irrespective of their age.

Influence of Medical Factors

With the elderly population increasing, the number of patients attending for dental care with extensive and complex medical histories is also increasing and this has many implications, not least how these medical conditions impact on the periodontium.

Varied drug therapies can impact in a number of ways, but this is a function of the medication the patient is taking rather than the patient's age. It is, however, a fact that older patients are highly likely to be taking medication. There are a number of drug therapies that can impact on the periodontium, and exacerbate periodontal disease. For example:

- Drug-induced gingival overgrowth associated with calcium channel-blocking drugs, antiepileptic drugs and cyclosprin used in transplant patients.
- Xerostomia, which can lead to root caries and plaque accumulation, is caused by a variety of drugs, including antidepressants, antihypertensives, or anxiolytics.

As well as issues related to the medical history, it is also important to remember that older patients may have issues regarding mobility and manual dexterity. With increasing age, patients may find difficulty attending for their dental care, and in fact a small number may need to be treated at home, which clearly compromises the range of treatments that can be offered. The issue of reduced manual dexterity is also important, and may lead to problems with maintaining a satisfactory level of oral hygiene, with the resulting impact on the periodontium. Given the recent research evidence for periodontal disease as a major putative risk factor for systemic disease, these factors increase the importance when treatment planning the elderly.

Attachment Loss

It is often thought that attachment loss is more frequently seen in older patients and this is indeed true, but it is not true to say that increasing age is a risk factor for periodontal disease. Individuals over 65 years exhibit more bone and attachment loss than younger individuals, but this is a result of progression of disease over a number of years rather than an increased susceptibility to disease in older age groups.

Gingival recession is frequently seen in older patients and may have a number of implications as far as patient management is concerned. It can lead to exposure of the root surface with an increased incidence of root caries (Fig 4-1), abrasion lesions and thermal sensitivity, all of which can be exacerbated in a patient suffering with xerostomia. Another important consequence is that gingival recession may expose root furcations in molar teeth, leading to an increase in plaque accumulation, which may result in problems with treatment and maintenance. It is important to note that treatment of periodontal disease, along with the disease process itself, can result in gingival recession and sensitivity. It is thus important to warn patients of such complications prior to undertaking periodontal therapy.

Research has shown conclusively that chronological ageing *per se* does not inevitably lead to periodontal disease associated attachment loss.

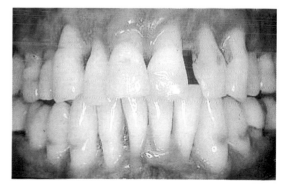

Fig 4-1 Gingival recession exposing root surfaces with root caries evident.

To summarise this section, a large variety of changes within the periodontal tissues has been identified in older subjects. Some of these changes are, however, controversial, and have not been demonstrated by all research groups. The histological, microbiological and biochemical changes, whilst interesting in themselves, may not have as dramatic an impact upon patient management as initially thought, and, for most practitioners, the key issue is how they relate to the clinical management of their patients. The next two sections will address these issues.

The Older Patient's Attitude to Periodontal Disease and its Management

As discussed above, the response of older patients to periodontal disease and its management is affected by a number of factors, which includes the individual subject's biological characteristics. There are psychosocial factors that impinge on the periodontal health of such patients. Such factors can influence a patient's behaviour. The most important of these is "self-efficacy". Self-efficacy can be regarded as giving the patient the belief that by changing their pattern of behaviour they can bring about a desired outcome. For example, if a patient practises a high standard of oral hygiene then this will reduce the risk of periodontal disease progression in that patient. Self-efficacy is strongly associated with health knowledge, attitudes and behaviour, which can produce improved health outcomes, and can be used as tools to target patients that are at risk of periodontal disease.

As far as periodontal disease and its treatment are concerned, older patients appear to respond in a manner similar to when they were younger. A number of studies have demonstrated that for the majority of adult life there is little change in intellect, and thus older patients are able to understand and act on any information given. However, health problems and biological decline can result in a reduction in the ability to perform certain tasks, such as a reduced ability to maintain a high standard of oral hygiene.

It is important to be aware that older patients are more prone to information overload, so the manner in which information is imparted is important, and the practitioner should aim to provide information in small doses with repeated reinforcement of the concepts involved.

The older patient may also be more likely to have experienced major life events, such as loss of a partner, divorce, etc., and such important life events may lead to the patient having low self-esteem. The diagnosis and management of peri-

odontal disease may, therefore, be low on their priority list, and they may be difficult to motivate in order to achieve a successful therapeutic outcome.
It has also been observed that the elderly more frequently experience depression, and the resulting medication used in its treatment may result in difficulty for the practitioner in motivating the patient. It should also be noted that antidepressant therapy can result in a reduction in salivary flow, which also has a significant impact on the oral health.

The Clinical Relevance of Age Changes to the Treatment of Periodontal Disease

For the practitioner the most important part of this chapter is how the changes previously discussed impinge on the day-to-day management of their patients. As with all patients, it is important that regular monitoring of the periodontal status is performed. This should include a Basic Periodontal Examination (BPE), as recommended by the British Society of Periodontology, at each recall appointment, along with an assessment of oral hygiene and instigation of appropriate treatment, where indicated. Whilst the BPE is a useful screen, it does not measure attachment loss and may underscore disease experience in older patients, who have recession and furcation involvement.

Assessment of plaque levels using a plaque score is a useful tool to monitor and motivate patients. Oral hygiene instruction is extremely important in all patients, but crucial in patients with periodontal disease, and, as with all oral hygiene instruction, it should be adapted and modified for each individual patient. This is particularly important in the elderly patient.

The following principles are useful in delivering the oral hygiene message:
- Discuss the concepts step-by-step.
- Avoid giving too much information at one time. Limited, frequent reinforcement is important.
- Encourage feedback and discuss the issues raised.
- Reinforce the spoken instruction with the use of diagrams and models, and use patient information sheets.
- Be realistic in what you are asking the patient to do.
- Older patients may have manual dexterity problems and the methods of brushing and interproximal cleaning should be adapted to overcome such problems.

For example, modifications to toothbrush handles to improve grip are useful. This can be achieved by the use of foam tubes, or simply by wrapping elastic bands around the handle of a standard toothbrush to aid its use (Fig 4-2). Cleaning of interproximal spaces is also important. A large range of interproximal brushes with conventional handles is currently available (Fig 4-3). It is also worth considering recommending the use of powered toothbrushes, which can aid plaque removal. The oscillation of the toothbrush head and wider handles can improve grip for the patient (Fig 4-4).

With all these oral hygiene issues, it is important carefully to demonstrate the techniques, and to ask the patient to try them in the dental surgery to ensure an appropriate technique is being used. Older patients will tend to have more restorations, which may compromise their oral hygiene. If a particular restoration is compromising oral hygiene, then consideration should be given as to whether a more hygienic restoration could be placed. Oral hygiene measures need to be targeted at the area of concern in order to reduce the levels of plaque accumulation.

As previously mentioned, gingival recession may be relatively common in

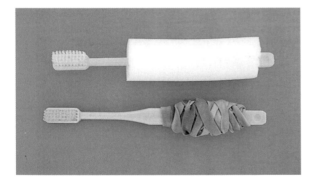

Fig 4-2 Two conventional toothbrushes modified to help patients with dexterity problems: (a) using elastic bands; (b) with foam handle.

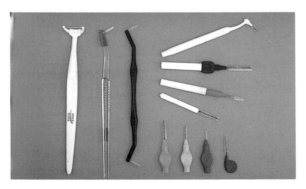

Fig 4-3 Range of interproximal cleaning aids.

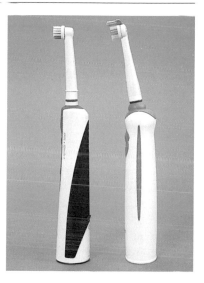

Fig 4-4 Electric toothbrushes. Thick handles aid grip.

older patients, and may predispose to root caries, so it is important to look closely at the patient's diet and reduce the levels and frequency of sugar intake. It may also be useful to consider the use of fluoride mouth rinses, or the application of topical fluoride to sites at risk of root caries.

Attachment loss can cause exposure of root furcations. This may result in the loss of vitality of pulpal tissue, because a direct communication to the pulp may occur when furcation canals are present. Thus, teeth with attachment loss exposing the furcation area should be regularly monitored for any signs of loss of vitality.

It is important to reinforce the concept that periodontal disease is not a consequence of age *per se*, but due to chronic exposure to risk factors over a number of years. In other words, the reason older people have more periodontal bone loss is because, in general, periodontal disease runs a slow chronic course, and thus attachment loss will be greater in older subjects. It is also important to remember that a proportion of older patients will have complex medical histories and be taking extensive medications, which may have an impact on the natural history of periodontal disease. If risk factors such as prolonged use of medication, smoking and denture wearing are excluded; the oral mucosa and periodontium in older patients have a similar appearance to those of younger subjects, and will respond to treatment in a similar manner.

Once treatment has been undertaken and a successful clinical outcome has been achieved, then the issue of maintenance needs to be considered, including risk assessment. (This applies to all patients, irrespective of age or whether they have experienced periodontal disease.)

In the patient treated for periodontitis this should include:
- amount of attachment loss
- plaque-retention factors (e.g. restorations, crowding, exposed furcations)
- patient motivation (level of oral hygiene)
- medical history
- manual dexterity
- smoking habits
- the treatment carried out.

By taking these factors into account, an informed judgement as to the period of patient recall can be determined. For patients with periodontitis a three-month recall is often suggested, but this can be modified depending on the factors listed above.

It is important to be aware that, although a number of features of the periodontium change with age, the same treatment modalities are appropriate in the management of periodontal disease in the adult elderly as are used in a younger patient, as long as the treatment planning recognises and treats the patient as an individual. The overall health care provision for adult elderly patients, and how this relates to their dental management, is also worthy of careful consideration.

Conclusions

- The population is living longer, with the proportion of patients over 65 years of age increasing. Additionally, patients are keeping more of their natural teeth, and their expectations of dental treatment are increasing.
- A large variety of age changes have been demonstrated in the periodontium, but these appear to have a small impact on periodontal disease progression and therapeutic outcomes.
- Periodontal disease, although seen more frequently in older subjects, is not part of the ageing process, but a consequence of disease progression in susceptible subjects over a number of years.
- Older patients may have social, medical and physical features that may impact on their periodontal condition, and these need to be taken into account in their management.

- In general, older patients will respond biologically to periodontal treatment as well as younger individuals, and thus the full range of periodontal therapies should be used in their treatment.

Further Reading

Smith DG and Seymour RA. Periodontal Disease and Treatment in the Elderly: 1. Dental Update 1989;6:18-24.

Smith DG and Seymour RA. Periodontal Disease and Treatment in the Elderly: 2 Dental Update 1989;7:50-55.

Wennstrom JL. Treatment of periodontal disease in older adults. Periodontology 2000, 1998;16:106 112.

Chapter 5

Root Caries: Aetiology, Diagnosis and Management

Aim

The aims of this chapter are to provide the practitioner with a review of the aetiology, diagnosis and management methodologies for root caries.

Outcome

The practitioner by the end of this chapter should be in a position to use an understanding of the aetiology and diagnosis of root caries to formulate contemporary treatment strategies for root caries.

Terminology

Dental caries is a disease of the mineralised tissues of teeth caused by the action of microorganisms on fermentable carbohydrates. It is characterised by demineralisation of the mineral portion of the tissues followed by the disintegration of the organic material.

Primary root carious lesions may be defined as lesions resulting from a carious attack initiating on root structure below the cemento-enamel junction (CEJ) with no initial involvement of the adjacent enamel or restorations. It can be arrested and remineralisation can occur.

Secondary root caries may be defined as lesions resulting from a carious attack on root structure adjacent to an existing restoration.

Epidemiology of Root Caries

In the older population, prevalence of root caries can vary between 57% and 88%. The greater prevalence is associated with the prolonged retention of teeth in older age groups and increased exposure of root surfaces, coupled with the ageing of the population. Incidence studies have shown that 30–40% of people studied develop root caries. Proximal surfaces may account for up to 54% of root carious lesions.

Aetiology

Root caries is a dynamic disease process with the potential for remineralisation as well as demineralisation to occur. A summary of the factors influencing the dynamics of root caries development is shown in Fig 5-1.

Host

Cementum comprises 50% organic and 50% inorganic material. Periodontal fibres called Sharpey's Fibres traverse it. Cementum exists in a cellular and an acellular form, with the cellular form covering the apical third of the root and the acellular cementum forming a thin layer adjacent to the dentine surface. Cementum is 150-200 mm wide apically but only 20-50 mm wide at the CEJ. In 10% of cases cementum does not reach as far coronally as the CEJ, exposing the underlying dentine. With ageing, there is increased exposure of root surfaces, and when exposure of the root surface occurs cementum is lost, especially on the facial surfaces, and dentine is exposed.

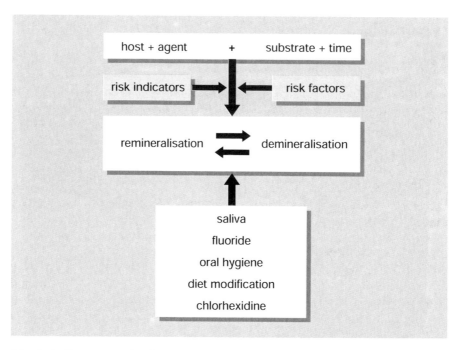

Fig 5-1 Factors involved in the demineralisation/remineralisation of root caries lesions.

Microorganisms

Various types of microorganisms have been associated with primary root caries, including mutans streptococci, non-mutans streptococci, gram-positive pleomorphic rods (GPPR), including Actinomyces spp. and lactobacilli.

Substrate

Development of root caries has been associated with those patients who give a diet history of more exposures to fermentable carbohydrate per week.

Time

For caries on the root surface to occur, the microorganisms metabolise the carbohydrates and acid is produced which can lead to demineralisation of the dental tissues. The disease process is dynamic, and remineralisation can occur as the pH rises above the critical value for cementum and dentine - pH 6.5. The longer the period that demineralisation is taking place the more likely it is that caries will develop. Consequently, factors that prolong the carious attack, such as xerostomia, repeated carbohydrate intake or partial-denture wearing, will increase the probability of dental decay developing.

Risk Factors and Risk Indicators

Based on epidemiological studies, a variety of risk factors and risk indicators have been determined. The risk factors and risk indicators can help identify individuals who are at increased risk of developing root caries. These are summarised in Table 5-1.

Diagnosis

Increased levels of microorganisms are associated with specific clinical characteristics of primary root caries lesions, namely:

- *Proximity to the gingival margin.* The closer a lesion is to the gingival margin the more likely it is to be active.
- *Texture.* Lesion texture (specifically lesion hardness as opposed to surface roughness) as a diagnostic criterion for root carious activity was validated when lesions which were categorised as soft on probing were shown to harbour the greatest number of bacteria associated with primary root caries activity.
- *Cavitation.* With increasing cavity depth lesion activity increases.
- *Size.* Larger lesions are more likely to be active than smaller lesions.

Table 5-1 Risk factors and risk indicators for root caries.

	Risk Indicators	Risk Factors
Sociodemographic	age education race institutionalisation gender decreased cognition	age race institutionalisation gender
Physical/medical	chronic diseases	anxiety level disability/recent illness
Intra-oral	Mutans streptococci Lactobacilli Candida albicans saliva flow rate	Lactobacilli
Environmental	systemic fluoride	systemic fluoride
Behavioural	regular check-ups emergency dental visit tobacco use carbohydrate intake infrequent tooth- brushing	social integration tobacco carbohydrate intake

Oral health status	poor oral hygiene
	gingivitis
	loss of attachment
	calculus
	gingival recession
	periodontal pockets
	  > 3 mm
	coronal caries experience
	root caries experience
	few remaining teeth
	partial denture
		poor oral hygiene
		gingivitis
		loss of attachment
		
		gingival recession
		periodontal pockets
		  > 3 mm
		coronal caries experience
		root caries experience
		few remaining teeth

Furthermore, special tests can aid in the diagnosis of root caries. Correctly angled bitewing radiographs have been shown to be useful in detecting mesial or distal root carious lesions, as are shown in Fig 5-2.

Management of Primary Root Caries Lesions

Rationale

The purposes of treatment of carious dentine are:

- To arrest the progress of the caries.
- If necessary, to promote healing of the remaining dentine and pulp.
- To restore the tooth to normal function.

Treatment should also:

- Be easy to execute so that reasonable levels of success can be achieved.
- Be cost effective so that patients can be treated without undue cost to themselves or society.
- Compensate for possible non-compliance with subsequent home therapy.

Treatment encompasses a range of modalities from preventive measures to removal of the carious tissue and restoration of the lesion. Identification of primary root caries lesions based on lesion activity (in effect, the relationship between the levels of microorganisms and the clinical characteristics) would be preferable to lesion identification based on disease history alone. Lesions that had been identified as active could be targeted for specific management, whilst inactive lesions would not be subjected to unnecessary treatment.

The activity of primary root caries lesions has led to the formulation of an

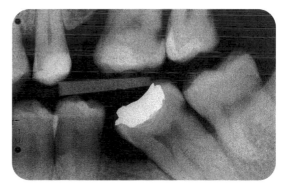

Fig 5-2 Bitewing radiograph showing proximal root caries distally on 27 and distally on 37.

Index of Perceived Treatment Need. The relationship between perceived treatment need of primary root caries lesions and their clinical characteristics is shown in Table 5-2.

After patient assessment, communication with the patient regarding their

Table 5-2 The relationship between perceived treatment need of primary root caries lesions and their clinical characteristics.

Clinical Characteristics	→	Perceived Treatment Need
Hard	→	No treatment
Leathery, small, easily cleansable and approaching a hard texture	→	Chemotherapy
Leathery, shallow, easily maintained, plaque-free	→	Caries debridement
All soft lesions	→	Caries debridement and restoration
Leathery, difficult to maintain, plaque-free.	→	Caries debridement and restoration
Large cavitated leathery lesions.	→	Caries debridement and restoration
Pulpal integrity at risk.	→	Caries debridement and restoration

disease status, contributing factors and treatment modalities comprise the most important phase of patient care. On the basis of disease activity, the following protocol for the treatment of root caries lesions can be applied.

Prevention

Provision of appropriate preventive care is desirable to prevent the development of primary root caries lesions.

Oral hygiene

Primary prevention of root caries involves prevention of periodontal disease and recession as well as the removal of plaque from the exposed root surfaces. A considerable degree of commitment and dexterity is required of the patient, which they may not be able to deliver.

Dietary counselling
The aim of dietary counselling is the reduction in the frequency and amount of refined carbohydrate intake.

Saliva stimulation
The anticaries effects of saliva include acid neutralisation, buffering and sugar clearance. It appears that the buffering capacity of saliva is of more relevance in caries prevention than a high flow rate. The relationship between buffering capacity and saliva flow rate is not linear and approaches a maximum at intermediate flow rates. Mastication such as chewing sugar-free gum can stimulate salivation.

Chemomechanical

Chemomechanical intervention should be considered for those lesions which are small, easily cleansable and leathery to hard texture. Such a regimen would serve to alter the balance of the carious process so that its progress is arrested. The main chemomechanical agents are fluoride and chlorhexidine.

Fluoride
Fluoride appears to act in preventing primary root caries by modifying the dynamics of the carious process either through its antimicrobial activity or by affecting the dental hard tissues. It can be delivered systemically or topically. Systemic water fluoridation has been shown to be associated with a reduced prevalence of primary root caries.

Most of the cariostatic effect of fluoride has been ascribed to its topical effect on the carious process in the oral cavity. Root surfaces significantly concentrate fluoride following topical fluoride treatment.

Chlorhexidine
Chlorhexidine is an antiseptic whith antimicrobial action based on its ability to affect the metabolism and structures of cariogenic microorganisms. The *in vivo* antimicrobial action of chlorhexidine is derived from the fact that teeth and mucosal surfaces adsorb it and it is subsequently released in a bac-

teriostatic concentration over a prolonged period of time.

There are several different vehicles for topical fluoride or chlorhexidine delivery, including mouth rinses, toothpastes, gels, chewing gum tablets and varnishes.

The optimum concentration of fluoride or chlorhexidine, the best delivery mechanism and the optimum frequency of application for root caries inhibition have yet to be developed. A problem with self-applied therapy is that it is dependent on patient compliance, so the use of varnishes has the benefit of being able to be applied to specific sites and has been shown to reduce the development of root caries lesions. Research has shown that application of a chlorhexidine varnish to exposed root surfaces at three-monthly intervals resulted in significantly fewer decayed and filled root surfaces compared to a control group.

Caries Debridement and Lesion Recontouring

This approach has been recommended for those lesions which are leathery, shallow, and readily maintained plaque-free, the rationale being that the root caries lesion can be recontoured using polishing burs until the surface is smooth and easily cleansable by the patient. Concern about this methodology has been expressed, as recontouring may result in a concave area that is plaque retentive. The base of the recontoured dentine is closer to the pulp and those root caries lesions that are located on proximal surfaces might not be accessible for instrumentation and chemomechanical management. Consequently, recontouring should be used on those lesions that are on surfaces that can be easily cleaned and closely monitored such as overdenture abutments and labial surfaces. In other circumstances restoration of the resulting defect after caries removal may be the most appropriate management option.

Whilst there may be some scope for future development of innovative treatment techniques for primary root caries lesions, conventional caries removal is still used.

Carious Dentine to be Removed and the Lesion Restored

Caries removal and restoration of the resulting defect is warranted in those lesions that are soft, for leathery lesions in surfaces judged to be difficult to maintain plaque-free, and for large, cavitated leathery lesions where pulpal integrity is thought to be at risk. Restorative management of primary root caries is a challenge because of the difficulties of visibility; moisture control and access to the lesions; proximity of the pulp; proximity to the gingival margin and the high organic content of the dentine. Several methods of caries removal may be considered.

Atraumatic restorative treatment

Atraumatic restorative treatment (ART) involves the removal of carious tissue using hand instruments and cavity restoration with a glass–ionomer cement. This has been carried out in single and multiple surfaces in the permanent dentition. Resin-modified glass–ionomer cements have been used to restore root caries lesions after caries removal with an excavator.

Chemomechanical caries removal

A recent development is the use of Carisolv™ (Medi-Team, Gothenburg, Sweden). This is a combination of 0.5% sodium hypochlorite and 0.1 M amino acids, glutamine, leucine and lysine. The manufacturers claim that the hypochlorite dissolves the decayed matter and the amino acids act as a buffer, protecting the healthy tissue. In vivo, Carisolv™ has been shown to be effective in caries removal. However, the mean time taken using Carisolv™ (10.62 min.) is more than twice as long as conventional caries removal (4.42 min.).

ART and chemomechanical management of root caries are easier for primary lesions and where access to the lesion is easy. Both ART and chemomechanical caries removal have the advantage over conventional caries removal in that there is little need for a handpiece, a reduced need for local anaesthesia and they can be used for domiciliary visits, especially ART (Figs 5-3, 5-4).

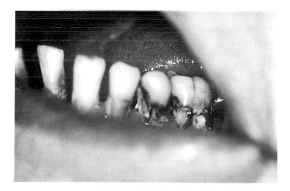

Fig 5-3 Root caries on 35 and 36 prior to ART in the patient's kitchen. (Courtesy of Dr C Dickinson)

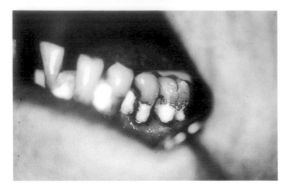

Fig 5-4 Root caries lesions on 35 and 36 after ART in patient's kitchen. (Courtesy of Dr C Dickinson)

Conventional caries removal: proximal and lingual lesions

Access to proximal lesions can present a challenge to the operator with respect to diagnosis and operative management, especially if the lesion lies in a furcal area. This may entail the removal of much healthy tissue to gain access to the lesion. Access may have to be gained via a buccal approach and it may be difficult to validate the efficacy of caries removal and restoration placement. This applies particularly for lower incisor teeth where removal of carious tissue from the approximal root surface has the potential to put the pulp at risk, the root dentine being very thin in this area.

Lingual lesions may also present an operative challenge owing to the presence of the tongue and the floor of the mouth (Fig 5-5). Such lesions can be associated in particular with poorly designed and maintained lower partial dentures (Fig 5-6).

Extension of the root caries lesion below the free margin of the gingiva or beyond the axial boundaries of the tooth may increase the difficulty in its restoration. It is difficult to remove excess material from marginal areas owing to irregularities on the root surface structure. Effective restoration may be very difficult to accomplish on an approximal surface or in an inaccessible furcal area.

The plastic materials available for the restoration of primary root caries lesions include amalgam, composite and glass-ionomer cement.

- Amalgam

As amalgam is mechanically retained, the creation of undercuts for retention may entail the sacrifice of sound tooth tissue. Amalgam cannot be used in areas where aesthetics are of prime importance. Whilst amalgam is easy to manipulate and its propensity to corrode at the tooth-amalgam interface

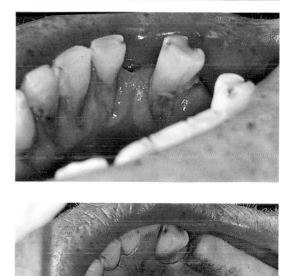

Fig 5-5 Lingual caries on 43 associated with poorly designed and maintained lower partial denture.

Fig 5-6 Poorly designed and maintained partial denture associated with lingual caries in Fig 5-5.

helps to reduce subsequent leakage, perfect marginal adaptation may be difficult to obtain, with the sequelae of leakage and secondary caries.

• Composite

Composite filling materials are superior to amalgams and glass-ionomer cements in terms of aesthetics but require careful handling to negate the effects of polymerisation shrinkage. Several steps are usually required to obtain a bond between composite and dentine and incremental filling is required to prevent composite resin shrinkage and subsequent gap formation.

Composites have no caries-preventive effects and post-operative sensitivity, discolouration and recurrent caries are often observed in root caries lesions restored with composite.

- Glass-ionomer cement

As glass-ionomer cements bonds chemically to enamel and dentine the need to extend cavity preparation is limited.

A major benefit of glass-ionomer cement is its ability to leach fluoride. The rate of fluoride release is not constant, with a large initial release rate, which gradually decreases. Glass-ionomer cements do have the ability to take up fluoride from topical sources and subsequently release fluoride at a higher rate. Levels of fluoride in plaque adjacent to glass-ionomer restorations have been found to be higher than those adjacent to composite resin materials.

Given its reasonable aesthetics, minimal leakage and conservative cavity preparation glass-ionomer cement is the material of choice for restoring root caries lesions.

Conclusions

- Root caries lesions on facial surfaces provide optimum access for non-invasive measures that can alter the dynamics of the disease process towards lesion remineralisation.
- Of particular concern is the finding from epidemiological studies that up to 54% of lesions may occur on proximal surfaces. These lesions are more difficult to diagnose and treat.
- Provision of care for primary root caries lesions based on perceived treatment need has led to a hierarchy of treatment strategies based on the activity of the lesions.
  -For the less severely affected lesions a strategy based on prevention coupled with a chemomechanical intervention may suffice.
  -At the other extreme, primary root caries lesions with a higher degree of activity have been treated using a surgical approach of excising the carious tissue and restoration of the resulting defect.
- Care for root caries lesions cannot be too prescriptive. Rather, it should focus on the patient so that optimum, appropriate care can be delivered.
- Patients identified as being at higher risk would benefit from more focused care, including more frequent recall to be cared for by their dental practitioner.

Further Reading

Beighton D, Lynch E, Heath MR. A microbiological study of primary root-caries lesions with different treatment needs. J Dent Res 1993;72:623-629.

Galan D, Lynch E. Epidemiology of root caries. Gerodontology 1993;10:59-71.

Seichter U. Root surface caries: a critical literature review. J Am Dent Assoc 1987; 115:305-310.

Chapter 6
Tooth Wear in Older Adults

Aim

The aim of this chapter is to discuss the cause of pathological tooth wear in older adults, its consequences and possible treatment options.

Outcome

At the end of this chapter, the practitioner should be familiar with the presenting signs of tooth wear and be able to diagnose the aetiological factors from the presenting signs. The practitioner should also recognise that, in older adults, intervention strategies should be as minimal as possible to reduce maintenance requirements.

Aetiology and Diagnosis

As older patients retain more teeth for life than ever before, a common finding is that of a worn dentition. The aetiology of tooth wear in this age group can be pathological or advanced physiological in origin. Tooth wear may not be problematic until the patient becomes concerned about:
- appearance
- function
- long-term prognosis for the remaining teeth
- comfort.

Tooth wear has a multifactorial aetiology. The causes of tooth surface loss are:
- *Attrition* – which can be defined as tooth wear caused by excessive tooth to tooth contact. A typical attritional pattern of tooth wear is shown in Fig 6-1. In this patient tooth wear of attritional aetiology is shared between the maxillary and mandibular teeth. This pattern of tooth wear is common in bruxists. *Attrition* may be suspected if the patient admits to grinding their teeth. A relative may also confirm that the patient may grind their teeth when asleep. The incisal and occlusal surfaces are flattened, and the maxillary and mandibular teeth coincide during excursive movements.

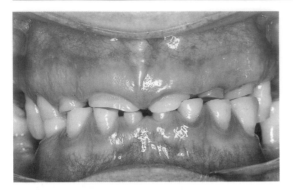

Fig 6-1 Typical pattern of tooth wear associated with attrition. Note the even contacts on the incisal edges of the anterior teeth.

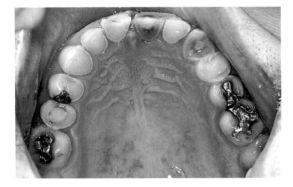

Fig 6-2 The dentition of a patient with erosive tooth wear of dietary origin. This patient consumed two litres of carbonated lemonade per day.

- *Erosion* – which can be defined as tooth wear caused by acid attack of the teeth not due to caries. Sources of the acid causing erosive lesions can be intrinsic (gastric origin) or extrinsic (e.g. of dietary origin or exposure to industrial acidic chemicals). A typical presentation of erosive tooth wear is shown in Fig 6-2. Erosion is characterised by a saucerised ("cupped-out") appearance of palatal and occlusal surfaces. The remaining enamel around the wear lesions is thin and often irregular. The teeth have a shiny appearance, but may appear stained if the wear process is not active. Amalgam restorations stand proud of the teeth. In severe cases, the labial and buccal aspects of the teeth may also be affected. Mandibular incisor teeth may be unaffected, and this is believed to be due to the tongue protecting these teeth. The distribution of the worn surfaces gives an indication of the aetiology of erosion. If erosion is caused by dietary factors alone, the palatal surfaces of maxillary anterior teeth are the most affected surfaces. Common causes of this type of erosion are carbonated drinks, citrus fruits and fruit juices consumed on a frequent basis. A dietary history should elicit these factors. Should lesions of an erosive aetiology be noticed on the molar teeth, the clinician should suspect that acid from the stomach is getting into the oral cavity. This type of tooth wear is seen in patients with:

-alcohol abuse behaviour
-hiatus hernia
-bulimia
-duodenal ulceration
-taking certain medications (e.g. ibuprofen).

In these situations, the dentist should consult with the patient's general medical practitioner. The diagnosis of tooth wear of erosive aetiology should be outlined to the medical practitioner. The dental practitioner should indicate that gastric reflux is the suspected cause, and enlist the aid of the medical practitioner in establishing a firm diagnosis. This may warrant referral to a gastroenterologist for further investigation.

• *Abrasion* – which can be defined as tooth wear caused by physical contact with an agent other than tooth (e.g. toothbrush abrasion) (Fig 6-3). Abra-

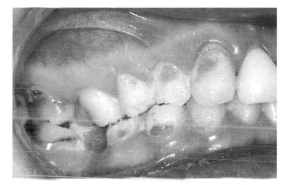

Fig 6-3 Abrasion of the buccal surfaces of teeth. This patient brushed with baking soda on a daily basis in an attempt to brighten the colour of her teeth.

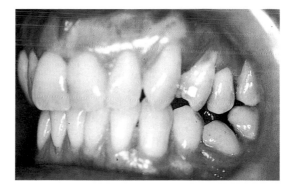

Fig 6-4 Tooth wear caused by heavy occlusal contacts (abfraction). Note the heavy contact between the buccal cusps of the premolar teeth. (Courtesy of Dr F Burke)

63

sion is characterised by a pattern of wear consistent with the tooth being abraded by an object such as a toothbrush. The affected surfaces, usually on the buccal and labial surfaces, will have irregular wear patterns.

- *Abfraction* – non-carious cervical tooth-surface loss caused by flexure of cusps. These present as wedge-shaped cavities on cervical margins of teeth and are typically found on maxillary canine and premolar teeth (Fig 6-4). It is difficult to envisage how this could be due to an abrasive agent such as a toothbrush, or why it is confined to a small number of teeth. The proposed mechanism for this is that occlusal stresses on teeth with steep cusps are transmitted to the cervical margin. The enamel in this region is thin, and consequently fractures.

Key Decisions

Tooth wear frequently has a multifactorial aetiology and management of tooth wear is complex. It can be difficult to decide whether tooth wear should be monitored once diagnosed or whether intervention is required. The key points in the management of tooth wear are summarised in Fig 6-5. Examine the pattern of wear on the tooth surfaces to diagnose the aetiology of tooth wear. The clinician should remember that it is not uncommon for more than one than one type of tooth wear to occur simultaneously.

The decision to intervene in tooth wear cases should be undertaken with care. If the patient is not in pain and has no functional or aesthetic complaints, then a preventive strategy and monitoring is advisable. In cases of attrition, an occlusal acrylic splint can be used for night-time wear to reduce tooth wear. When erosion is suspected, the precise cause should be investigated. A dietary history should be recorded, and possible erosive agents identified. The patient should be advised to modify the intake of erosive agents, specifically to reduce frequency of intake. If a gastric cause is suspected, then the patient's medical history should be reviewed and causes of gastric acid reflux identified. Occasionally, erosive tooth wear may be the first clue as to an underlying gastrointestinal disease. A further cause may be bulimia, although this is unusual in older adults. Appropriate medication and advice should be provided via the patient's physician. When abrasion is suspected, then the patient must be advised to modify their habits such as use of abrasive tooth cleaning agents. Where abfraction lesions are diagnosed, modification of occlusal contacts may be indicated.

When adopting a preventive approach, the clinician should be mindful of the threat to the vitality of the pulp. Simple intervention using direct composite resin restorations may be necessary if the wear process threatens pulp

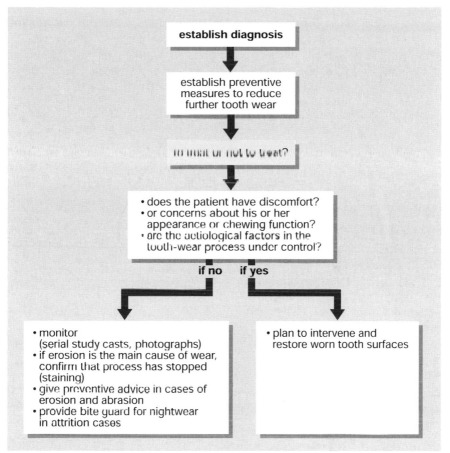

Fig 6-5 Key points in the management of tooth wear.

vitality. If the patient is unhappy with the appearance of their teeth or has sensitivity, then further intervention is warranted. A number of developments have increased the options for the management of tooth wear in older adults. Traditionally, full-mouth rehabilitation, including the use of crown-lengthening surgery and full veneer crown restorations were the mainstays of management of tooth wear. The extensive nature of these forms of treatment often proved a barrier to reconstruction of worn dentitions in the elderly, and removable options were more frequently used. In recent years, bonding to dentine has improved considerably, and bonded restorations are now more predictable and suitable for elderly patients.

Management of Tooth Wear

The various possible intervention strategies are outlined in Fig 6-6. When making a decision as to which of these strategies to employ, the following should be considered.

Is there adequate space for restorations?

If the wear process has proceeded rapidly, then there is usually plenty of space to place restorations without significantly increasing occlusal face height. However, as is frequently the case, the process is slow and there is compensatory downgrowth of the alveolus in an attempt to maintain face height. This leaves very little, if any, space for restorations. This situation is often encountered in erosion cases in the anterior dentition. The options available for creating space are:

- Restoring the teeth at an increased occlusal vertical dimension. This option is frequently used in older adults and involves restoring the occlu-

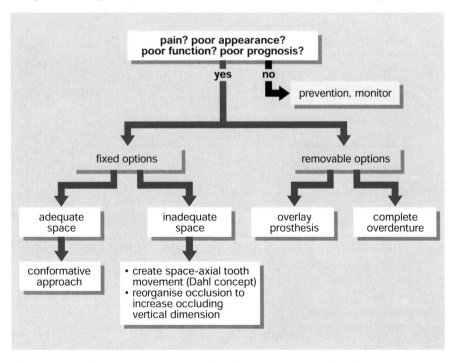

Fig 6-6 Possible treatment strategies for the management of tooth wear.

sal surfaces of the remaining teeth with fixed restorations or removable prostheses. Removable prostheses are indicated in severe wear cases or when teeth are missing. It is not clear how much opening of the vertical dimension a patient can tolerate, but most patients appear to tolerate increases of 4-6 mm. The clinician may assess tolerance of an increase in occlusal face height using an occlusal splint prior to definitive restorations, but this is not always necessary.

- Axial movement of teeth using the Dahl concept. This can be very effective in creating localised space for restorations, particularly on the anterior maxillary teeth. The technique involves placing restorations on the surfaces of anterior maxillary teeth that cause separation of the posterior teeth. A combination of intrusion of the teeth with restorations and over-eruption of the separated teeth creates space for restorations (Fig 6-7a,b). Dahl originally described the concept using a cast nickel-chrome alloy restorations cemented to the palatal aspects of maxillary incisor teeth in the management of localised anterior tooth wear. This restoration was left in place for periods of six to eight months or until the desired space was

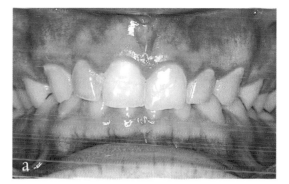

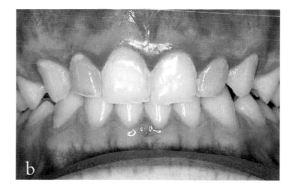

Fig 6-7 Space creation in an anterior tooth wear case using the Dahl concept: (a) at initial presentation; (b) following 8 months wearing a Dahl appliance. Note the decreased overbite.

created. When the appliance was removed, the posterior teeth had re-established contact and created room anteriorly for restorations. Composite resin restorations can also be used as an alternative to the traditional Dahl appliance. This approach will only work when posterior teeth are present in both arches. A further consideration is that tooth movement is unpredictable and detailed research into the use of this technique in older adults is lacking.

Fixed restorations

Adhesive restorations are widely used in the management of cervical tooth wear. Composite resin restorations offer the possibility of excellent aesthetics and good abrasion resistance. Glass–ionomer materials can also be used. These have excellent bonding properties and have the added advantage of leaching fluoride into the surrounding dentine. In cases at risk of caries, this can be a significant advantage. Disadvantages of glass-ionomers include poor abrasion resistance and appearance compared with composite resins. Resin-modified glass ionomers and compomers are further alternatives combining the desirable properties of both composite resins and glass-ionomers.

In terms of occlusal tooth wear, whether fixed restorations can be used depends on (a) the amount of remaining tooth structure when cemented restorations are chosen and (b) the availability of suitable bonding substrate if bonded restorative materials are chosen. Fixed restorations are preferred for minor to moderate tooth wear. The improvement in bonding restorative materials to dentine has enhanced the options for restoring minor-to-moderate degrees of tooth wear (i.e. wear not extending into the pulp). Restorative materials that can be used in this situation are:
1. composite resins (direct or indirect)
2. porcelains
3. non-precious metal alloys (nickel-chrome alloy)
4. precious metal alloys (Type III gold alloy).

For composite resin materials, very little tooth preparation is required. They are indicated when aesthetic requirements are paramount and have the advantage of being easy to repair. A disadvantage with composite is the potential for wear, and in severe bruxists they are unlikely to survive. They can be very effective in erosion cases. Diagnostic etching should be undertaken to see if the restoration can be bonded to enamel and dentine (Fig 6-8). Restorations bonded to dentine only have a much poorer retention rate and confidence in bonding is increased when a ring of etched enamel is visible. Sharp areas of enamel should be removed and the teeth isolated using a rubber dam.

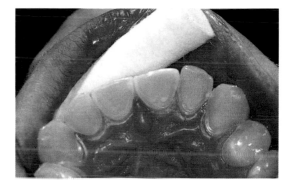

Fig 6-8 Diagnostic etching to assess amount of enamel present. When a rim of enamel is identified around the periphery of the tooth, confidence in bonding is increased.

Using a bonding system of choice the clinician should then directly bond composite resin to the worn tooth surfaces. Care should be taken to follow the manufacturer's instructions when applying bonding resins, as failure to do so will compromise bond strength. Sufficient bulk of composite (around 2 mm in thickness) should be placed to avoid breakage of the material when in function.

Porcelain arguably has the best aesthetic qualities. This may be essential if the restoration involves the incisal edge of an anterior tooth or if the incisal edge is translucent. Unlike composite resin restorations, a micromechanical bond to tooth structure is possible with ceramic restorations and there is some evidence that higher bond strengths are therefore possible. A number of porcelain systems are currently available – namely, traditional feldspathic porcelain, pressable ceramics (e.g. Empress-2) and, infiltrated ceramics (e.g. InCeram). Feldspathic porcelain has excellent aesthetic properties but relatively poor flexural strength. Pressable and infiltrated ceramics use high-strength cores to substantially increase flexural strength. These cores are then veneered with feldspathic porcelain to achieve an aesthetic restoration. Feldspathic and pressable ceramics can be bonded or cemented to the tooth. Infiltrated ceramics cannot be etched and therefore must be cemented to the tooth.

The margins of the prepared tooth must be carefully finished to avoid setting up excessive stresses that may lead to fracture of the porcelain. If traditional porcelain materials are used, then approximately 1mm of space is required. If high-strength porcelain systems such as InCeram or Procera are used, then 1.5-2 mm of space is required as these materials have a core material veneered with feldspathic porcelain. The occluding surface of the porcelain must be highly polished to avoid abrasion of the opposing tooth surface.

The fitting surface of the porcelain should be etched with hydrofluoric acid gel, preferably at the chairside, and a silane primer should also be applied. The restoration should then be bonded onto the tooth use a composite luting cement, taking care to ensure that the restoration is fully seated. A potential disadvantage with porcelain restorations is they are not easy to repair in the case of fracture.

Non-precious metal alloy such as nickel chromium has proved to be very useful in resin-bonded bridgework. These materials are relatively inexpensive and very durable in the oral environment. Tooth reduction of approximately 0.75 mm should be made to allow adequate thickness of metal. The fitting surface of the metal restoration should be sandblasted using aluminium oxide particles (50 microns) prior to fitting the restoration to increase bond strength. The restoration should then be cemented using cement with a high affinity for oxidised metal, such as 4 - META. This form of restoration is indicated in cases of attrition and when aesthetic requirements are not paramount.

Precious metal alloy such as Type III gold alloy may also be used. The tooth preparation is similar to that of preparations required for non-precious metal alloy. These materials are easier to adjust than non-precious metals. They are more expensive than non-precious metal alloys, and this could be significant in the older adult. Bonding to precious metal alloys is not as strong as non-precious alloys, as there is very little formation of oxide layer and oxide layers are not as well achieved using sandblasting. Heat-treating the fitting surface (400° C for four minutes in a laboratory furnace) increases oxide layer formation and improves bond strength.

Indications for a removable prosthesis

In some tooth wear cases, insufficient tooth structure remains to retain fixed prostheses, and it is not possible to provide extra tooth structure using crown-lengthening periodontal surgery. Some patients may also have missing teeth and require tooth replacement as well as treatment of worn teeth. In situations such as that shown in Fig 6-9, it is possible to improve appearance and function using an overlay removable prosthesis. This design of prosthesis utilises the remaining natural dentition to retain a removable prosthesis in the same manner as an RPD. The bases for these prostheses can be made of acrylic resin or cobalt-chromium metal alloy and the overlay material can be acrylic resin or metal. Acrylic resin has the advantage of being easy to adjust and repair, but may not be very durable. This is particularly relevant in cases of attrition.

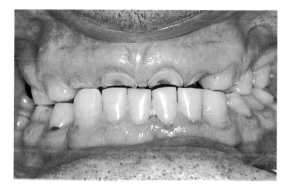

Fig 6-9 Insufficient tooth structure remains for fixed restorations. The patient was treated using a removable prosthesis.

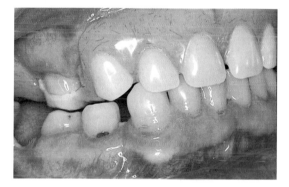

Fig 6-10 Restoration of appearance and function in a patient with severe tooth wear of erosive aetiology. Simple acrylic removable overlay appliance.

Planning overlay prostheses

There are a number of decisions to make at this stage:

- Is the first prosthesis to be an interim or definitive prosthesis?
- Are all worn teeth to be retained?
- How much should the occluding vertical dimension be increased?

In most cases of advanced tooth wear that have progressed untreated, it is unlikely that the patient will have worn a denture. The clinician may decide to use a simple acrylic overlay denture to test the patient's tolerance of a removable prosthesis (Fig 6-10). A further consideration when making this decision is whether a period of tissue healing is required. It is possible that some teeth may have worn down to gingival level, and these teeth may need to be extracted.

The clinician should decide by how much the occluding vertical dimension should be increased. A key influence on this decision is the desired appearance.

Overlay prostheses: clinical stages

- Remedial treatment to treat caries and periodontal disease should be undertaken. Once the dentition is stable, the clinician can then provide an overlay prosthesis.
- Primary impressions should be made using either irreversible hydrocolloid or elastomeric impression materials. The resultant model should then be surveyed to indicate a suitable path of insertion for the overlay denture. This procedure should indicate the undercuts on the teeth and the bony undercuts. Using this information, the clinician should design a path of insertion and direct retention features such as clasps. It may also be desirable to create metal backings for the teeth, as these may help prevent fracture of the denture teeth. Backings are particularly indicated where there is a lack of interocclusal space.
- Prior to recording the final impressions, some preparation of the teeth is required. These include rest seats, guide planes and creation of undercuts for direct retainers. Teeth that will be covered by the denture should have any sharp edges removed and finish lines should be placed on the labial surfaces of these teeth to indicate where the acrylic resin should finish. This will also help blend the tooth–coloured acrylic resin with the teeth to improve aesthetics. Final impressions should be recorded in a customised impression tray using irreversible hydrocolloid or elastomeric impression material. If a metal-based onlay denture is used, then a metal framework tryin procedure is required.
- The jaw relationship should be registered using the desired amount of visible tooth with the lips at rest as a guide. Wax should be added to the rim in the area overlying the teeth until the desired level is reached.
- At the next stage, a trial denture should be used to verify the occlusal contacts and appearance. Once these have been verified as correct, the clinician should then proceed on to the delivery stage. The working cast should be checked to ensure that unwanted undercuts have been blocked out – failure to do this could lead to difficulties inserting the denture.
- At the delivery stage, the patient should be instructed how to insert and remove the overlay denture. Post insertion instructions, including cleaning instructions, should be given to the patient and a review appointment arranged.

Conclusions

- Tooth wear is often multifactorial in aetiology, and may be difficult to treat. It is not always necessary to intervene.
- In cases of erosion, the dental practitioner may need to liaise with the patient's medical practitioner to determine the cause of acid reflux into the oral cavity.
- Preventive measures should be emphasised, and any treatment intervention should be as minimally invasive as possible.
- Removable and fixed options can be used in the treatment of tooth wear. Improved bonding of materials to dentine has increased the range of possibilities for fixed restorations in the management of tooth wear.

Further Reading

Summitt JB, Robbins JW, Schwartz, RS, dos Santos J. Fundamentals of Operative Dentistry: A Contemporary Approach. 2nd Ed. Chicago: Quintessence, 2001.

Chapter 7
Endodontics and the Older Adult

Aim

To consider special issues affecting endodontic decision-making and treatment in the elderly.

Outcome

At the end of this chapter, the practitioner should have raised awareness of general and local factors that may support or undermine the case for root canal treatment in an elderly patient.

Endodontics and the Older Adult

Apical periodontitis has the same aetiology in all age groups – namely, microbial infection of the pulp space. Tissue responses to infection control are predictable, and there is no reason to expect that the elderly will respond any less well to adequate treatment than other age groups. The decision whether to extract a pulpally or periapically involved tooth in the elderly should not therefore be based on age considerations, but on an evaluation of general and local factors for and against tooth preservation. Some of these will be of special relevance in the elderly.

Key Issues

Can the tooth be saved?
Is root canal treatment technically possible, and will the tooth be restorable after treatment?

Should the tooth be saved?
Even if the tooth can be root canal treated and restored, is there any benefit to be gained by its preservation? Would retention or loss of the tooth create general or local complications in patient care?

Can the Tooth be Saved?

Is the tooth restorable?

Teeth judged after clinical and radiographic examination to be unrestorable should be extracted. There are no rewards for heroically conducting root canal treatment on teeth that have no functional capacity due to tissue loss, fracture or periodontal compromise.

Can infection be controlled?

Predictable treatment demands an access to the infected pulp space. If this is complicated by limited mouth opening; unfavourable tooth alignment or overeruption; intolerance of lengthy operative procedures or calcification of the pulp space, it may not be possible to save the tooth, and treatment should be planned accordingly.

Will the patient consent to treatment?

Treatment planning should not be self-indulgent and go beyond the realistic aspirations of the patient. There may be occasions when patients will not consent or subject themselves to complex treatment plans, ruling out the preservation of a tooth that could be saved by root canal treatment.

Is the proposed care affordable?

Ideal treatment plans are all well and good, but these are sometimes beyond the financial means of patients. Simpler treatment is often dictated, and, once again, a tooth that could be preserved should be sacrificed within a simpler plan of care.

Should the Tooth be Saved?

Medical considerations

There are few medical contraindications to endodontic therapy. Antibiotic prophylaxis is not usually required for endodontic treatment confined to the pulp space since this carries a very low risk of significant bacteraemia. In fact, root canal treatment may be positively indicated to avoid extraction in patients with cardiac problems or those taking anticoagulant medication.

Relative contraindications to endodontic treatment include:
- Patients requiring *radiotherapy* to the head and neck region. All foci of infection should be removed prior to commencement of radiotherapy.
- *Poor compliance* (e.g. patients with Parkinson's disease, tremors, or dementia).

- Patients *unable to lie comfortably in a dental chair* for prolonged periods (e.g. those with ankylosing spondylitis).

Is this a critical tooth?

The functional and aesthetic value of the tooth should be reviewed. From a functional point of view, the tooth may not be critical and extraction may be a more attractive option. Conversely, the tooth may be useful as a retainer for an RPD (Fig 7-1) or as an overdenture abutment.

- Teeth that are periodontally compromised may serve well as overdenture abutments after root canal treatment and decoronation.
- Retention of a final standing molar may help to preserve occlusal stability, avoid the need for an RPD altogether, or at least avoid the need for it to have a free-end saddle.
- Even short-term retention of a tooth may facilitate the progressive transition into edentulousness by providing natural occlusal stops and facilitating the development of motor skills in controlling partial dentures.

On the negative side, an awkwardly positioned tooth which is destabilising an opposing prosthesis or interfering with reconstruction should not be preserved for its own sake.

Endodontic Challenges for the "Old" Tooth

Assessment and diagnosis

In common with other age groups, most pulp and periapical disease in the elderly is painless. If pain is present, a standard pain history should provide clues on its origin (pulpal or periapical) and location. Symptoms should be

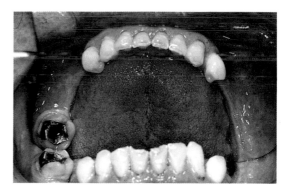

Fig 7-1 Lone-standing molar tooth which is non vital. Loss of this tooth would make tolerance of a removable partial denture less likely. Endodontic treatment of this critical tooth should be seriously considered.

reproduced by standard pulp sensitivity (thermal and electrical stimulation) and periapical (percussion sensitivity) tests.

Pulp-sensitivity testing is often inconclusive in heavily restored teeth, and those with fibrosed or calcified pulps. Ice sticks provide an intense and durable thermal challenge and can be especially useful to stimulate older teeth. Electronic pulp testers provide no qualitative information on pulp status, but may add to the evidence that a pulp is dead. However, negative thermal and even electrical pulp testing do not necessarily denote a non-vital tooth in need of extraction or root canal treatment. Other circumstantial evidence of pulp condition may come from the presence of:
- caries
- large and fractured restorations
- tooth fractures
- soft-tissue swelling and discharge.

Good-quality periapical radiographs provide essential supplementary evidence of coronal, pulpal and periapical condition.

All of this information should be drawn upon to build a picture of pulp/periapical status and the need for operative intervention. This information will also be tempered by the nature of the reconstruction planned.

Differential Diagnosis

Clinicians should be alert to the occasional lesion which appears unusual, including primary and metastatic tumours, and take account of other conditions in their differential pain diagnosis, including:

- Atypical Facial Pain
- cracked cusp syndrome
- post-herpetic neuralgia.

PerioEndo Lesions

Elderly dentitions are likely to display some degree of periodontal and periapical disease. Lesions are usually distinct and easy to manage by conventional means. Occasionally, localised areas of deep probing, suppuration, mobility and radiographic bone loss are encountered which present diagnostic and treatment planning dilemmas.

Primary endodontic lesions

Purulent lesions of endodontic origin can discharge through the periodontal ligament or gingivae to give the appearance of a periodontal pocket. The probing defect is usually deep (often to the apex) and narrow, and accompanied by a pulp which is unresponsive to thermal and electrical challenge. Root planing will not close the defect and will destroy attachment apparatus. Root-canal treatment will restore the tissues to normal, with closure of the sinus within days of canal preparation.

Primary periodontal lesions

Purulent periodontal lesions are usually encountered within the context of general periodontal involvement. The pulp responds to thermal and electrical challenge, and the defect is a broad pocket, usually with subgingival calculus present. Endodontic treatment will not heal the lesion. Healing will only follow thorough periodontal care.

Combined lesions

Here, there is a non-vital pulp and discharge of endodontic origin through the periodontium in addition to marginal periodontal bone loss. It is usually impossible to discern how much of the deepened probing, bone loss, mobility and discharge are due to each of the lesions. Any tissue damage due to endodontic disease will heal completely after root-canal treatment that is able to control intracanal infection. On the other hand, periodontal treatment will provide little or no bone regeneration, and healing only with a long junctional epithelium. It is consequently important to heal all of the destruction due to endodontic disease before potentially destroying attachment by over-extended periodontal instrumentation.

The regenerating endodontic treatment is, therefore, done first, with periodontal care confined to oral hygiene instruction and scaling until the outcome of endodontic treatment is known (approximately three months). Non-surgical periodontal treatment can then be employed to manage any residual disease of periodontal origin.

Problems of Access to Infection

Pulps undergo physiological and reactive changes as patients age. Changes are not, however, uniform, and are not necessarily concentrated in the chronologically old. Pulp canals in the elderly are not necessarily narrow and difficult to manage, and reactive changes in the young and middle-aged can be equally, or more, challenging.

Key Changes Which May Compromise Infection Control in the Pulp Space

Increased fibrosis

As the pulp ages, it becomes less cellular and more fibrotic. The tissue is tougher and may not be penetrated as easily with files. The risk this presents is that entry even to a seemingly large pulp results in compaction of pulp tissue to form a dense collagenous plug that is as impregnable as any calcified deposit. There is special merit in the elderly of removing pulp tissue with barbed broaches and the routine use of lubricants to allow instruments to glide through tissue rather than compacting it.

Diminution of pulp space

Physiological age changes reduce the height of pulp horns; make the pulp shrink out of the crown of anterior teeth; reduce the distance between chamber roof and floor in posterior teeth; and cause the pulp to narrow concentrically in roots. Although these changes are considered physiological, it is a consistent finding that apical canal diameters remain wide into old age, suggesting a reactive element.

Changes considered truly reactive include irregular, irritation dentine deposits, laid down to wall off tubules opened by caries, trauma, operative dentistry, wear and periodontal disease.

Obliteration with irregular calcification

The diminishing pulp space can be complicated by the growth of irregular calcifications around degenerating blood vessels and nerve cells. These changes usually comprise spheroidal "pulp stones" in the coronal chamber, and linear deposits with a "grain" and texture like a wet cocktail stick in the canals. Radiographs may suggest that these changes completely obliterate the pulp space, but they are usually interspersed with soft tissue fronds that provide space and nutrition for microbial infection, whilst easing the path for operative disruption and entry.

Notes on the Safe Pulp Access in "Old" Teeth

- Do not assume that the elderly are insensitive. Give local anaesthetic for endodontic access.
- Orientate the access bur against a good-quality preoperative radiograph to confirm the depth and position of the pulp.

- Orientate line and depth during access preparation – and keep checking.
- Optimise vision with good light, magnification, a front-silvered mirror, and a long DG16 canal probe to explore the chamber.
- If there is concern about losing alignment, leave the rubber dam off until the chamber is entered.
- Clear mineralised deposits from the interior of the pulp chamber with an ultrasonic scaler.
- Work to locate the dark, domed floor of the pulp chamber with its network of fissures that will guide to canal entrances.
- Check all bleeding spots with an electronic apex locator before assuming they are canals and opening them widely. Repair perforations immediately.

Probe all canal entrances and feel the probe stick before picking up files. If there is no "stick", there is no path for files to follow. Chase canal entrances with small, narrow-shanked burs (e.g. Goose neck bur) and probe the cocktail stick-like contents again until a stick is felt. You then have a path to follow.

- Lubricate the chamber and walk into the canals with small files (#10 or lower) and a watch-winding/picking motion. As the constricted canal entrance opens, the file will often drop into the wider apical reaches.
- Once negotiated, there are generally few special difficulties or differences in the root canal treatment of older teeth.
- Old teeth and their surrounding tissues will respond as well to infection control as any other.
- If progress is not made, or infection control is otherwise compromised, a decision should be made to:

- Leave the canal untreated, especially if the tooth is not a critical tooth and no expensive reconstruction is planned. Best evidence suggests a risk of approximately 50% of teeth with apical periodontitis becoming painful in a 10-year period. Conversely, concerns are currently arising on the systemic consequences of chronic inflammatory lesions of dental origin.

- Refer for root canal treatment.

- Extract the tooth.

Decisions on the course of action should only be made on the basis of properly informed patient consent.

Conclusions

- Age is not a barrier to root canal treatment; tissues respond well to infection control at any age.
- Root canal treatment is not necessarily difficult in the elderly.

- Decision-making on the preservation or loss of pulpally involved teeth should be based on a thorough evaluation of general and local factors.
- There may be especially compelling reasons to lose or preserve teeth in the elderly.

Further Reading

Cohen S, Burns RC (Eds.) Pathways of the Pulp. 8th ed. St Louis: Mosby, 2002.

Chapter 8
Functionally Oriented Treatment Planning

Aim

The aim of this chapter is to describe the principles of the shortened dental arch concept

Outcome

At the end of this chapter, the reader should be aware that it is not always necessary to replace all missing teeth. The decision to replace teeth should be based on whether prosthetic replacement will improve function, appearance and comfort. Limiting treatment goals to provide functional rather than a complete dentition is becoming acceptable in light of recent research findings.

Do We Need to Replace all Missing Teeth?

In many cases, patient and dentist opinion differs on what sort of dental treatment is required. This disparity between professionally assessed treatment need and patient demand is particularly apparent in older patients. When a patient presents with missing teeth, the clinician should consider the following:

1. Does the patient have any problems chewing food?
2. Does the patient have any appearance or cosmetic concerns arising from the missing teeth?
3. Does the patient have any discomfort arising from the missing teeth?
4. Is there any evidence of occlusal instability as a result of the missing teeth?

If the answer to any one of these questions is "yes", then there is a good case to be made for replacing the missing teeth. If the answer to all of these questions is "no", then replacing the missing teeth is not necessary. Population-based studies indicate that patients not sufficiently motivated to use RPDs decline to wear them. A common finding from these studies is that missing posterior teeth are not always considered a problem by patients. However, patients are often persuaded to seek replacement of teeth when anterior teeth are lost. They may feel compelled to wear an RPD to replace both anterior and posterior missing teeth when their primary concern is the anterior tooth space, and this may be a source of dissatisfaction.

A further consideration is the issue of biological price – does the potential benefit of providing a prosthesis outweigh the potential damage it may cause to the remainder of the natural dentition? RPDs are associated with high levels of dental caries and periodontal disease, particularly in patients who have inadequate oral hygiene measures. Conventional fixed bridgework may involve extensive tooth preparations that may damage the vitality of the retainer teeth.

Older adults often have differing functional needs to younger adults, and do not always require a fully intact dentition to have adequate oral function. As adults gradually lose teeth, they have the capability to adapt to the limitations this imposes. Patients who have adapted well to tooth loss are unlikely to seek treatment to replace missing teeth unless anterior teeth are lost. A further consideration is the ability of an older adult to undertake a long course of treatment. Frail patients or those with chronic debilitating illness may be unable to accept prolonged courses of treatment and more modest treatment goals should be established.

Influences on Tooth Replacement Decisions

The clinician must determine the following when considering treatment options to replace missing teeth:
- Patient's motivation – their previous dental history will give an indication of compliance.
- Finance – how much is the patient willing to pay for dental treatment?
- Ability to attend for treatment.

Possible treatment options for replacing missing teeth in partially dentate patients are shown in Fig 8-1. Highly motivated patients are likely to seek tooth replacement, and this is indicated when the patient has satisfactory plaque control procedures. They should also be willing to attend for numerous appointments and be able to finance complex treatment. Some patients may not be able to afford expensive treatment, or be willing to attend for numerous visits for dental treatment. Modest treatment goals should be established for these patients and this may involve limitation of treatment goals to provide a functional rather than a complete dentition.

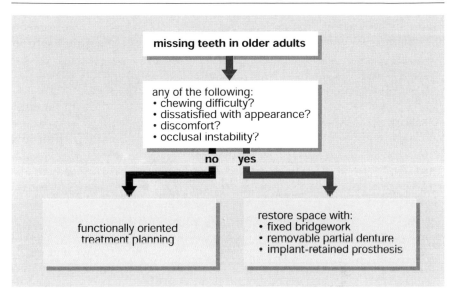

Fig 8-1 Possible treatment options for the replacement of missing teeth in older adults.

The Shortened Dental Arch Concept

Rationale

Many epidemiological studies have indicated that older adults do not always seek treatment to replace missing posterior teeth. Further researchers have suggested that older patients have differing functional needs to younger adults and may not need treatment to replace all missing teeth. A final consideration is that financial resources for dental treatment are diminishing, and dentists will increasingly have to think strategically about long-term treatment goals. Kayser and co-workers proposed the shortened dental arch (SDA) concept as a means of limiting treatment goals to provide a functional rather than a complete dentition. This concept is underpinned by directing treatment resources at preserving the anterior and premolar teeth. They identified these teeth as strategic teeth, or teeth considered important to the patient. Posterior teeth are replaced if they are likely to improve function, comfort or aesthetics.

Indications/contraindications to shortened dental arches

The *indications* for SDA are:
1. Caries and periodontal disease mainly confined to the posterior teeth.
2. There is a favourable prognosis for the anterior and premolar teeth.

85

3. Limited financial resources for dental care.

These criteria are rather broad, but essentially mean that there must be a good prognosis for the anterior and premolar teeth if this treatment strategy is going to work. This is intended to be a lifelong strategy and not a short-term stop-gap. Loss of teeth in shortened dental arches may lead to a complete change of treatment strategy.

SDA is considered to be contraindicated if:
1. There is a pre-existing temporomandibular joint dysfunction.
2. There are signs of pathological tooth wear.
3. The patient has a significant dentoalveolar malrelationship.
4. The patient is under the age of 45 years.
5. There is a poor prognosis for the remaining dentition, specifically advanced periodontal disease.

In the past it was believed that impaired chewing function, occlusal instability and temporomandibular joint problems were inevitable consequences of tooth loss. This is simply not the case in all patients. Patients have the ability to adapt to tooth loss, and as long as sufficient numbers of occluding pairs of teeth remain, chewing ability is not necessarily affected adversely. Temporomandibular joint disorders have a multifactorial aetiology, and not simply a direct result of tooth loss. When a patient with a reduced dentition presents with TMD, it is possible that the reduced number of occluding units is an aetiological factor. These patients should then receive treatment to increase the number of occluding units either with an RPD or implant-retained prostheses as part of the rehabilitation of TMD.

The presence of pathological tooth wear or advanced periodontal disease indicates that the long-term prognosis of the dentition is uncertain and therefore the SDA approach is contraindicated. In Figs 8-2 and 8-3, the patients had shortened dental arches and the remaining teeth had signs of pathological tooth wear and occlusal instability. These teeth had a poor long-term prognosis, and the SDA approach would not be indicated. A key element in the success of SDA is the maintenance of at least three occluding pairs of posterior teeth. In the case of dento-alveolar malrelationship, it is unlikely that this can be achieved and therefore SDA is unlikely to achieve satisfactory function. Finally, there is no definite lower age limit for using the SDA approach. It is felt that the presence of posterior teeth is important to the development of the stomatognathic system in adults under the age of 45 years, and therefore treatment to replace missing posterior teeth should be undertaken.

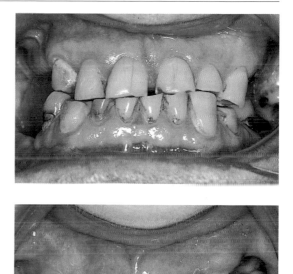

Fig 8-2 Evidence of pathological tooth wear in the remaining dentition. Application of the shortened dental arch concept is contraindicated due to the poor long-term prognosis for these teeth.

Fig 8-3 Patient with a grossly unstable occlusion. Shortened dental arch therapy is contraindicated.

A number of studies have indicated that a shortened dental arch can provide satisfactory oral function in carefully selected patients. The patient in Fig 8-4 has had missing posterior teeth for many years. He has not altered his diet, and does not want to have these missing posterior teeth replaced. His occlusion has remained stable, and the long-term prognosis is good.

When the only teeth remaining in a shortened dental arch are the incisor and canine teeth, it is unlikely that this number of teeth will provide satisfactory function. A further potential problem is that the remaining teeth may start to drift as they become overloaded. Furthermore, when a mandibular dentition shortened to this number of teeth opposes a maxillary complete removable denture, replacement of the maxillary alveolar ridge with flabby tissue is a common consequence. The complete replacement denture is often unstable and unretentive in this situation without the use of a mandibular RPD to provide posterior occluding contacts.

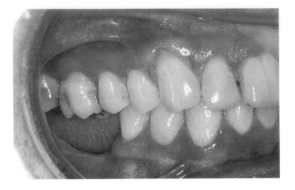

Fig 8-4 Patient with missing mandibular molars. This patient had lost his molar teeth many years previously. Note the stability of the maxillary occlusal plane.

Applications of the SDA Concept

Ideally, a premolar dentition would be the end-point of the SDA approach. This would involve maintaining occlusal contacts from second premolar to second premolar with intact maxillary and mandibular dentitions. However, this is an unusual clinical situation. More common clinical situations encountered are an edentulous maxillary arch opposed by a shortened mandibular dental arch, or shortened arches that are not intact (Fig 8-5).

In the case of a shortened dental arch opposed by an edentulous arch, the clinician has the option of maintaining a shortened dental arch or providing an RPD. The argument against free-end saddle RPDs is their potential for causing damage to the surrounding natural dentition. However, they may help to stabilise an opposing complete denture. This should be considered if the edentate arch is severely resorbed or if there is evidence of a flabby ridge. In this situation, the anterior maxillary ridge moves beneath the denture during function thus causing it to become displaced. If the only occluding contacts are on anterior mandibular teeth, this is likely to exacerbate the situation. Management of the partially dentate mandibular arch against an edentulous maxillary arch consists of the following:

- If the mandibular arch is reduced to the canine and incisor teeth, then plan to use a mandibular RPD. If first premolar teeth are present, then use either an RPD or extend the shortened dental arches with fixed bridgework. Once the treatment plan has been made, record primary impressions.
- If the anterior maxillary ridge is flabby, then care should be taken to avoid displacing the ridge when making the master impression. A mucostatic technique using impression plaster or two-stage technique using impression paste and plaster in a customised tray with a window in the region of

the flabby tissue should be used. Impressions for an RPD should be recorded in elastomer or irreversible hydrocolloid (alginate).

- At the jaw relationship registration stage, a facebow transfer should be recorded. This will allow the technician to set denture teeth for a trial denture on a semi-adjustable articulator. This will facilitate the setting up of denture teeth in balanced occlusion and articulation.
- Verify the adequacy of the trial dentures.
- Insert denture. Minor occlusal adjustments can be made at chairside.

A further option would be to refine the occlusion using a clinical remount procedure. This is done by recording a precentric occlusal record and remounting the dentures on a semi-adjustable articulator. The occlusion of the dentures can then be refined and returned to the clinic for delivery. If the shortened dental arch is reduced to the first premolar teeth, then extension of the arch can be achieved using either cantilevered bridgework or implant-retained crowns. When using cantilevered bridgework, a single unit

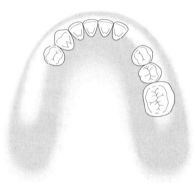

Fig 8-5 Shortened dental arch that is not intact. Teeth 35, 36, 37, 43 and 47 are missing. Tooth spaces 35 and 43 could be restored using fixed bridgework.

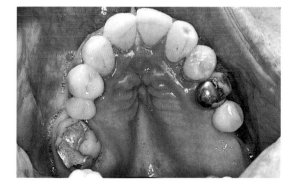

Fig 8-6 Extension of a shortened dental arch using cantilevered, resin-bonded bridgework, with 25 as the retainer. Note the use of a small pontic.

on either side or both sides of the dental arch can be added (Fig 8-6). The pontic should not be any bigger than the retainer to avoid occlusal overload. Options for bridgework include conventional, full-coverage retainers constructed in porcelain-fused-to-metal or resin-bonded bridgework of Maryland design.

Conventional retainers are indicated if the abutment tooth is heavily restored. If abutment teeth are unrestored, or minimally restored, resin-bonded bridgework may be indicated. If this treatment option is chosen, the abutment teeth should be prepared to make the bridgework mechanically retentive. Principle design features in this treatment modality are:
1. 180° wrap-around of the metalwork on the abutment tooth; 0.5 mm reduction of enamel.
2. Proximal grooves.
3. Occlusal support using rest seats prepared on the mesial and distal occlusal surface.
4. Supragingival finish lines in enamel.

These features are shown diagrammatically in Fig 8-7. Care must be taken to ensure that the pontic is not in heavy contact with opposing teeth during excursive movements, as this is likely to cause failure.

Current research indicates that this approach works well in older adults, and provides satisfactory oral function. Significantly, in this older age group, retention of plaque is reduced and this helps preserve the remainder of the natural dentition. Where the shortened dental arches are not intact, then these tooth spaces should be restored by bridgework if possible. If this is not

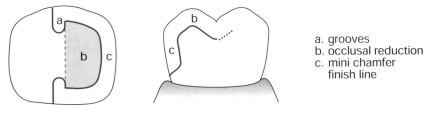

Occlusal view   Buccal view

a. grooves
b. occlusal reduction
c. mini chamfer
   finish line

Fig 8-7 Preparation features for posterior resin-bonded bridges. Incorporation of these features increases the success rate of this treatment modality.

possible, then the SDA approach may not be indicated. Implant-retained crowns may also be used to extend shortened dental arches. This approach has the advantage of not involving preparation of natural teeth. However, the disadvantages of this approach are:
• Prolonged treatment time.
• Surgery is required to place implants.
• Relatively expensive treatment modality.

In situations where the dental arch has been reduced to the canine and incisor teeth, RPDs may not have been tolerated. A dentition reduced to this extent is unlikely to provide adequate oral function, and the only way to increase the size of the occlusal table would be to provide implant retained crowns in the premolar region. Age is not a contraindication for dental implants, but the clinician should consider if the patient is fit for surgery to place implants. A further concern has been that functional overload may cause failure of osseointegration in this situation. The occlusal scheme must be carefully designed to reduce this risk, and the clinician should also consider the possibility of using wide diameter implants.

Final Considerations

When considering whether to limit treatment to maintaining shortened dental arches, it is essential that the prognosis for the reminder of the natural dentition is reasonable. There are a number of potential drawbacks to employing this treatment strategy. In avoiding the use of an RPD, the tongue can migrate into the posterior tooth spaces (Fig 8-8). Should further teeth be lost and an RPD be required, there may be too little space for denture teeth. The patient will also not have the opportunity to learn how to adapt

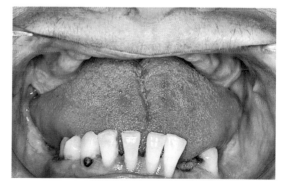

Fig 8-8 Migration of the tongue into posterior tooth spaces, with resultant loss of the neutral zone. This causes major difficulties in the provision of a removable partial denture.

to wearing a removable prosthesis. If more teeth are lost the patient may not be able to adapt to wearing a removable denture, particularly if tooth loss occurs late in life. Despite this, shortened dental arches appear to provide a satisfactory level of oral function and offer a predictable treatment option in carefully selected older adults.

Conclusions

- Older adults may not need to have all missing teeth replaced.
- The anterior and premolar teeth are critical teeth in terms of function and appearance. Limiting treatment goals to maintain these teeth may be acceptable in older adults.
- Application of the shortened dental arch (SDA) concept provides satisfactory oral function in carefully selected adults.

Further Reading

Owall B, Kayser AF, Carlsson GE. Prosthodontics: Principles and Management Strategies. St Louis: Mosby, 1995.

Chapter 9
Tooth Replacement in Partially Dentate Older Adults

Aim

As adults are retaining teeth into old age, the requirement for complete replacement dentures will decrease. This chapter aims to describe how decisions can be made regarding tooth replacement in older adults.

Outcome

At the end of this chapter, the practitioner should appreciate that some older adults will seek treatment to replace missing teeth. Fixed and removable prostheses can restore function, appearance and occlusal stability following tooth loss. The practitioner should also understand that poor maintenance of RPDs is associated with high levels of dental disease and that care must be taken to avoid further tooth loss. Preparation of abutments to receive bridge retainers may also endanger the vitality of the teeth and margins of retainers are susceptible to dental caries. The concept of "biological price" should also be understood.

Planning Tooth Replacement

RPDs are one of the most widely used prostheses to replace missing teeth. In this chapter, issues that are particular to the elderly are raised. As was discussed in Chapter 8, it is not always essential to replace missing teeth. Nonetheless, there are a number of clinical situations where some form of prosthesis is required to replace teeth. In older patients, a minimum of twenty teeth is usually required for adequate chewing function. Once the complement of teeth falls below this threshold, chewing ability may diminish to an unsatisfactory level. Should anterior teeth be lost, research indicates that patients are very likely to seek treatment to replace missing teeth. Speech is also affected by loss of teeth, particularly anterior teeth.

Occlusal instability may also occur after loss of teeth. This is manifested in drifting of teeth into adjacent tooth spaces and/or over-eruption of teeth in

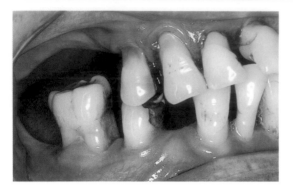

Fig 9-1 Occlusal instability following the loss of teeth, with drifting of maxillary anterior teeth.

the opposing arch (Fig 9-1). A further potential consequence of occlusal overloading is drifting of anterior teeth in a buccal direction. This is particularly likely if the anterior teeth have had a significant amount of bone loss.

When deciding whether to provide a prosthesis, the clinician must decide if the "biological price" is worth paying. Any prosthesis may potentially compromise oral health – RPDs are associated with increased levels of plaque and fixed prostheses require removal of tooth structure during preparation. If the need to replace teeth is deemed essential, then the biological price may be worth paying.

Fixed or Removable Prostheses?

There are a number of factors to consider when deciding whether to use fixed or removable prostheses to replace missing teeth. The outcome of this decision-making process depends on local and general factors.

Long spans
As a general rule, the risk of failure of fixed bridgework increases when more than two teeth are replaced. This is particularly the case when teeth in the canine or first premolar tooth region are replaced using anterior and premolar teeth. Lateral incisor teeth are regarded as poor-quality retainer teeth as they have short roots and small clinical crowns. A further problem with long-span bridgework is the potential for fracture of the porcelain on porcelain-fused-to-metal bridgework. Precious or semiprecious metal alloy is more flexible than porcelain and consequently when a long span bridge flexes in function, porcelain may fracture. RPDs do not have the same problems and may be more appropriate in longspan situations.

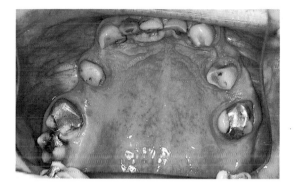

Fig 9-2 Removable partial dentures can simultaneously replace many teeth, as in this patient.

Number of tooth spaces (saddle areas)

As an RPD can replace a number of teeth simultaneously, they are indicated in situations where there are multiple tooth spaces (Fig 9-2). It is possible to use multiple bridges when tooth spaces are small, but this is time consuming and may not be acceptable to the patient.

Soft tissue profile

When teeth have been lost due to trauma, the associated tissues can also be lost. A similar clinical picture can be seen when severe resorption occurs. As well as occlusogingival resorption, bucco–palatal resorption can also occur (Fig 9-3). Replacement of teeth and tissue with a fixed prosthesis can be very difficult, and it may lead to an unsatisfactory aesthetic result (Fig 9-4). The pontic teeth may look very long compared with the retainer teeth. A removable acrylic flange can be constructed to replace resorbed bone and this is placed above the pontics. However, food stagnation is often a problem in such situations. An RPD may be a better option for replacing large amounts of soft tissue, and possibilities should be carefully discussed with the dental technician. The acrylic flange on the denture can be contoured in such a way as to compensate for loss of soft tissue, and a very satisfactory aesthetic result may be achieved (Fig 9-5).

Status of potential abutment teeth

When heavily restored abutment teeth are present, the clinician has to consider what would happen in the event of problems with these teeth. Particular concern arises with teeth that have had endodontic treatment. These are high-risk teeth for failure as bridge abutments and may compromise the entire prosthesis. It may be preferable to use a removable prosthesis if the prognosis of abutment teeth is questionable. If the prognosis is considered favourable, then both fixed and removable prostheses are indicated. Should

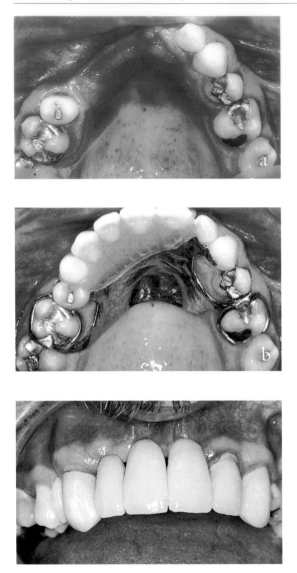

Fig 9-3 Loss of bone as well as teeth occurred following trauma in this patient. Note: (a) the degree of bone loss on the labial aspect of the alveolar ridge; (b) how this is replaced by the removable partial denture. (Courtesy of Dr N Jepson)

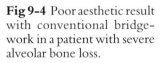

Fig 9-4 Poor aesthetic result with conventional bridgework in a patient with severe alveolar bone loss.

an RPD be the prosthesis of choice, then heavily restored abutment teeth could have full coverage crown restorations that incorporate features such as rest seats and guide planes (Fig 9-6). The preparation of the teeth in these situations is a little more extensive to allow room for features to be incorporated in the crowns. If surveyed features are planned, then it is essential that design features of the RPD be considered prior to construction of the

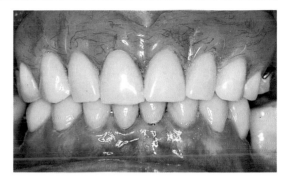

Fig 9-5 Satisfactory cosmetic result achieved with a removable partial denture in a patient with severe alveolar bone loss.

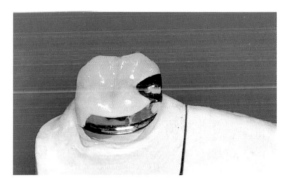

Fig 9-6 Milled rest seats and guide surfaces incorporated into full coverage crowns for patient provided with a removable partial denture.

crowns. A cast of the patient's teeth should be surveyed and the position of rest, clasps, guide surfaces and connectors planned. This will indicate the ideal position for rest seats, guide planes and undercuts on subsequent full coverage crowns.

Patient preference
As with any form of dental treatment, the patient's wishes must be carefully considered. The various treatment options should be discussed in detail with the patient, including advantages and disadvantages. The long-term maintenance requirements must also be carefully discussed. Although a fixed prosthesis may be possible, elderly patients may prefer a less invasive option and choose a removable prosthesis.

Fixed Prostheses in Older Adults: Special Considerations

Should fixed bridgework be chosen, further considerations in older adults include:

97

- Condition of potential abutment teeth.
- Patient ability to maintain satisfactory plaque control.

General principles of assessment and treatment planning should be followed and whole mouth care, not just care for an isolated tooth space, should be planned. Of particular relevance is the health of the gingivae, as inflamed gingival tissues make it difficult to record accurate working impressions. The occlusion should be checked for evidence of heavy guiding contacts and interocclusal space assessed. Guiding contacts on bridge pontics must be avoided. Occlusal surface wear or a history of repeated fracture of teeth or restorations indicates parafunction and lack of guidance during excursive movements. Failure to recognise and address these problems could compromise a fixed-bridge restoration. The vitality of abutment teeth should be checked, particularly heavily restored teeth. Teeth that have been endodontically treated are high-risk abutment teeth, owing to the possibility of tooth fracture or reinfection of the root canal system. A decision should be made as to whether old restorations should be replaced. A further consideration is the height of the crowns of potential abutment teeth. In older adults with moderate physiological tooth wear, the abutment teeth may be short and crown-lengthening periodontal surgery procedures may be required. As previously mentioned, design of fixed bridgework should facilitate plaque control, especially pontic design.

Implant-retained prostheses may also be considered. Age is not a contraindication to dental implants, and offers a number of advantages. Implant-retained prostheses do not rely on the natural dentition for retention and have a very good success rate. As with fixed bridgework, whole mouth care is essential. The health of the natural dentition and periodontal tissues should be assessed, as the natural dentition should be stable at the time of placing dental implants. Loss of natural teeth soon after completion of implant therapy is likely to compromise the implant-retained prosthesis. Parafunction may contraindicate implant-retained prostheses, as occlusal overload is a cause of delayed implant failure.

Surgery is required to place the implants and occasionally onlay bone grafting must precede this. Fear of surgery may discourage the patient from having this form of treatment, but careful explanation with the aid of photographs may be helpful. A further possibility is to introduce the patient to someone who has already been provided with an implant-retained prosthesis. They are also a relatively expensive restoration to provide, but this may be offset by the long-term stability this type of restoration offers when compared with removable options.

RPDs in Older Adults: Special Considerations

Standard design principles should be employed when providing RPDs for older adults. In this section, some situations commonly encountered in older adults are discussed further, specifically:
- Problems of the unbounded saddle.
- Reduced interocclusal space.
- Methods of direct retention.
- Maintenance issues.

Unbounded (free-end) saddles

In older adults, a common clinical presentation is that of the unbounded saddle (unilateral or bilateral). There is a differential of support for a prosthesis in this situation, and the denture will tend to rotate around an axis defined by the clasps (Fig 9-7). This will exert a torque force on the abutment teeth adjacent to the saddle area. Further clinical considerations include:
1. Path of insertion. As they are unbounded, it is relatively easy for the denture to fall out. If possible, a path of insertion that is different from the path of natural displacement should be designed.
2. Differential support for the denture between the teeth at one end and the soft tissues on the other. This causes the denture to sink into the tissues under occlusal load and exerts a torque force on the abutment teeth.
3. Horizontal movement. This can be reduced by proper extension of the flanges of the denture.

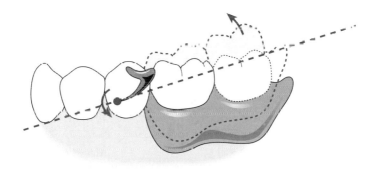

Fig 9-7 Axis of rotation about the abutment teeth in a bilateral free-end saddle removable partial denture.

4. Indirect retention. The denture will tend to move away from the tissues when chewing sticky food. The axis of rotation is around the clasp axis, and placing a component on the opposite side of the axis can reduce this.

Given the number of difficulties presented, it should not be surprising that compliance with wearing RPDs containing free-end saddles is variable. Studies of RPDs suggest that approximately 20-40% of these dentures are never worn or only used occasionally. The following section outlines some techniques that may reduce the difficulty with free-end saddle RPDs. Commonly used strategies in the management of the unbounded saddle to reduce sinking of the denture and torque forces on abutment teeth include:

- the RPI system of clasp design
- the altered–cast impression technique
- reduction of the occlusal table.

The RPI system of clasp design is designed to reduce torque force exerted on abutment teeth. The rest seat is placed on the mesial surface of the tooth. A guide plate is placed on the distal surface of the abutment tooth along the planned path of insertion. This should extend onto the lingual surface of the tooth to provide reciprocation for the clasp. In this system of design, the clasp is a gingivally approaching I-bar design. These design features are shown in Fig 9-8. This system of design should reduce torque forces on the abutment teeth.

The altered cast impression technique involves constructing the saddles of the denture using a muco-compressive impression technique. Once the

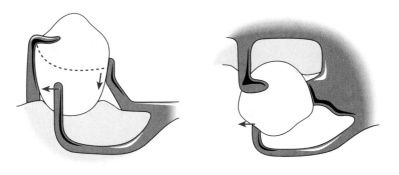

Buccal view   Occlusal view

Fig 9-8 Features of the RPI system of clasp design: rest seat on the mesial surface, proximal plate on the distal surface, and gingivally approaching I bar clasp.

framework has been constructed and fits adequately, the dental technician is instructed to place close-fitting acrylic trays on the saddle area of the framework. When these are returned to the clinician, impression material is placed into the saddles, and the framework seated in the mouth. Impression materials used for this purpose include impression wax or Zinc Oxide Eugenol paste. As the trays are close fitting, the material exerts a compressive force on the underlying tissues. The framework should be held in place using the rests, and digital pressure should not be exerted on the saddles. Once the impressions have been checked and deemed adequate, they are returned to the technician. The technician will then remove the saddle areas from the master cast, place the framework onto the cast and pour stone into the saddle areas. This creates an "altered cast" (Fig 9-9) that represents the tissues in a compressed state, and the saddle areas will be processed on this cast. The technique is particularly indicated when:

- there are more than two teeth missing in an unbounded saddle
- there has been significant resorption of the alveolar ridge.

Furthermore, this approach is only required in mandibular saddles, as the palate provides sufficient support in the maxilla to prevent sinking of the RPD under occlusal load.

Minimising the occlusal table can reduce occlusal forces. This can be achieved by using a smaller mould of tooth or fewer teeth. This should reduce forces generated into the soft tissues and theoretically should decrease resorption of the bony ridge.

Lack of Interocclusal Space

Once teeth are extracted, adjacent or opposing teeth may drift into the resid-

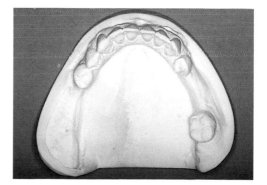

Fig 9-9 Altered cast prepared following use of a mucocompressive impression technique.

ual tooth space. This may lead to lack of space for replacement teeth if construction of a replacement prosthesis is delayed. When there is a reduction in space for restorations, care must be taken not to increase the occluding vertical dimension of occlusion using the RPDs alone (Fig 9-10). This will direct all the occlusal forces into the underlying tissues leading to discomfort. Any treatment intervention should keep the natural dentition in contact using a conformative or reorganisation approach. The possible options would be:

Conformative approach
- Do not replace all missing teeth.
- Use smaller teeth or occlude on the base plate.
- Use metal backings on the denture teeth.

Reorganisation approach
- Increase occluding vertical dimension using the denture teeth and onlays on the RPDs – metal or acrylic (Fig 9-11).

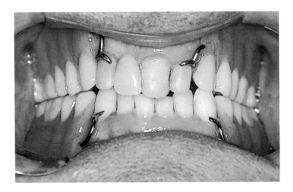

Fig 9-10 Excessive increase in occluding vertical dimension using bilateral free-end saddle removable partial dentures. This patient was unable to tolerate the dentures due to pain in the underlying ridges.

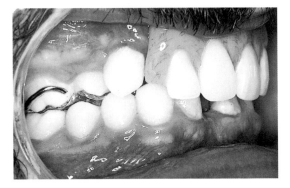

Fig 9-11 Use of onlay denture to achieve an increase in occluding vertical dimension using natural teeth and soft tissues.

102

In some cases, there simply is not enough space at the existing occluding vertical dimension to replace missing teeth, and not replacing all the teeth, or planning to occlude on the base plate is the treatment of choice. Sometimes, particularly in Kennedy Class IV situations, the use of metal backings is the treatment of choice. The normal grid mechanism for attaching denture teeth to the base plate takes up a lot of room, and to avoid increasing the occluding vertical dimension, the acrylic is left very thin. Potentially, this could lead to fracture of the acrylic and loss of teeth from the denture. An alternative is to extend the major connector of the denture into the saddle area as a "backing" for the denture teeth, thus avoiding the need for a grid attachment mechanism (Fig 9-12.) When planning to use metal backings, the clinician should determine acceptable denture tooth position in advance of constructing the framework using either an impression of the previous denture or a trial wax tooth set-up. Failure to do this could lead to difficulty in achieving satisfactory appearance.

Using a reorganised approach, onlays are used to increase the occluding vertical dimension by a planned amount and denture teeth occlude with other denture teeth or natural teeth at this new occluding face height.

This treatment strategy involves:
- Metal onlays. These are durable, but difficult to cast and adjust.
- Acrylic onlays. Easy to adjust, but not very durable and can be difficult to colour match with natural teeth.
- Combination of removable dentures and fixed restorations on natural teeth at the increased occluding vertical dimension.

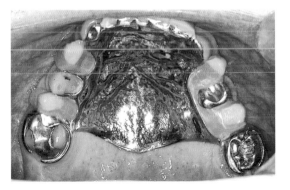

Fig 9-12 Use of metal backings for anterior teeth to prevent fracture of anterior saddle when inter-occlusal space is limited.

Methods of Direct Retention

Clasp retained

Clasps provide an effective means of retaining RPDs. Where possible they should be placed so as not to affect aesthetics. Further considerations include:

- *Length.* They should not be too short as this increases the rigidity of the clasp and can cause clasp fracture.
- *Clasp material.* Cobalt chromium alloy is commonly used and suitable for undercuts less than 0.25 mm in depth. Should the undercut depth be between 0.25 and 0.5 mm, cobalt chromium alloy clasps can be made more flexible by increasing their length. This will also make the clasp more prone to distortion. Once the undercut depth exceeds 0.5 mm, a material with a high modulus of elasticity such as gold alloy should be used.
- *Clasp position.* Clasp tips should not be placed too close to the gingival margin and if possible should not cover the root surface.

Precision attachment retained

A precision attachment can be extracoronal or intracoronal. They are designed to improve retention of the RPD and may be more acceptable cosmetically than clasps. Mechanisms of attachment can be via bars, press studs, magnets or dovetail and slots. The practitioner has to consider whether the potential benefit of having precision attachments outweighs the financial cost and complexity involved in providing them. Particular clinical problems with precision attachments include:

- They exert lateral forces on roots of teeth that may accelerate progress of periodontal attachment loss or cause root fracture.
- Extensive tooth preparations may be required to provide intracoronal attachments.
- They require a lot of space, and care must be taken not to weaken the denture by using large precision attachments.

Nonetheless, they may provide valuable means of retaining a denture in unfavourable situations like the one shown in Fig 9-13. This patient has a repaired cleft palate, and retention of his previous partial denture was unsatisfactory. By using a Rothermann attachment on tooth 23, significant improvement in retention was achieved.

Maintenance

Plaque control is complicated by the presence of an RPD, and this coupled with reduced manual dexterity in the elderly can potentially hasten tooth

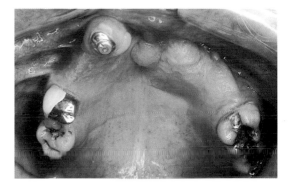

Fig 9-13 Patient with a cleft palate and a lone-standing anterior tooth. Use of a Rothermann precision attachment significantly improved the retention of his removable partial denture. (Courtesy of Mr F Nohl)

loss. It is therefore critical that homecare procedures are emphasised and monitored by the clinician. In terms of cleaning, the following procedures are recommended:

• The patient must be shown how to clean both natural teeth and the RPD. The advice should be repeated and emphasised to ensure that it is understood. Toothbrushes may need to be modified where manual dexterity is a problem. Further aids such as tufted interproximal toothbrushes or electric toothbrushes are useful. Older patients may struggle with dental floss, so be wary of recommending this without ensuring that the patient can use it.

• Toothpaste or hard bristle toothbrushes should not be used on the denture as these cause scratching of acrylic resin.

• Denture cleaners are also to be recommended, but the patient should be advised not to use cleaners that contain sodium hypochlorite (e.g. Milton) with metal-based dentures as these cause corrosion of the metal. The patient should also be encouraged to remove the denture when asleep.

Reline/rebase

The patient should be encouraged to attend for review appointments on a regular basis. It may be appropriate, especially in free-end saddle dentures, to consider reline or rebase procedures to reduce trauma to the denture-bearing area. Some teeth may gradually lose periodontal support, and the RPD should be modified to add these teeth when required.

Conclusions

• Whole mouth care is essential when planning tooth replacement in partially dentate patients.

105

- RPDs can be used to replace missing teeth when a patient has chewing difficulties, appearance concerns, discomfort or occlusal instability related to missing teeth.
- Fixed prostheses retained on teeth or implants can be used in older adults and should be planned using standard design and technique principles.
- Fixed and removable prostheses should be designed and constructed to be as tissue-friendly as possible. Provision of prostheses to replace missing teeth increases maintenance requirements.
- Poorly maintained RPDs are associated with high levels of dental disease. Regular review of patients with RPDs is recommended.

Further Reading

Davenport JC, Basker RM, Heath JR, Ralph JR, Glantz P-O, Hammond P. A Clinical Guide to Removable Partial Dentures. London: Macmillan, 2000.

Chapter 10

Overdentures: The Bottom Line for Older Adults?

Aim

This chapter aims to review the rationale for the use of complete overdentures in older adults.

Outcome

At the end of this chapter, the practitioner should be aware of the advantages and disadvantages of overdentures, the treatment of patients requiring overdentures and maintenance issues. The possibility of minimising bone loss and thus potentially overcoming some of the limitations of complete replacement dentures should also be recognised.

Rationale for Overdenture Therapy

This technique utilises roots of natural teeth to support a complete denture. Atrophy of alveolar bone occurs following the loss of natural teeth. This phenomenon is particularly noticeable in the mandible that resorbs at approximately four times the rate of resorption of alveolar bone in the maxilla. Transmission of masticatory forces to the underlying bone via the teeth is thought to provide a functional stimulus to the bone, thus leading to turnover of bone. Loss of teeth removes this stimulus and bone atrophy is the inevitable consequence. Despite extensive research, the reason for great individual variation in bone loss remains unclear. From the evidence currently available, it seems that post-extraction alveolar bone loss is influenced by a combination of both local and systemic factors. While the pathogenesis of alveolar bone loss remains unclear, there is no reliable way in which to predict the rate of alveolar bone loss on an individual basis.

During the 1970s, the technique of using roots of teeth to support removable complete dentures (overdentures) was described. Research at that time indicated that retention of roots beneath removable dentures maintained bone height and prevented alveolar bone resorption adjacent to the roots (see Fig 1-2). This greatly facilitated the stability and retention of complete dentures.

In some patients, the loss of most of the natural dentition may be inevitable. Given that complete replacement dentures have many limitations, a sensible "bottom line" in the management of older adults should be the retention of some roots to support complete overdentures.

Benefits of overdentures
Potential *benefits* of overdentures include:
* preservation of alveolar bone
* aiding the stability and retention of dentures
* psychological well-being
* maintaining proprioception.

In addition to preserving bone, the roots provide a means of increasing retention and stability of a complete denture. The contact between the roots themselves and the fitting surface of the denture provides a degree of friction grip. Furthermore, the roots can be used to retain precision attachments (Fig 10-1), which in turn can be used to enhance denture retention in certain situations.

Retention of some part of the natural dentition can be important from a psychological point of view for some patients. As the oral health of older adults improves, it seems likely that older adults will be less likely to accept that tooth loss is an inevitable part of the ageing process. Consequently, retaining some portion of their natural dentition will be of benefit.

Proprioceptive receptors are found in the periodontal ligaments of teeth and

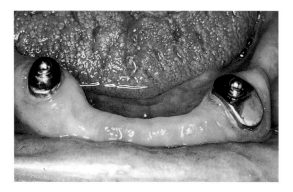

Fig 10-1 Ball attachments on cast post and diaphragm on mandibular overdenture abutments. Corresponding o-ring attachments are incorporated into the denture.

form part of the reflex loop for mastication. Masticatory forces are detected by these receptors and this information is conducted to the masticatory centre in the brain. A reflex loop is completed by signals being transmitted to the masticatory muscle groups in the jaw to depress the mandible. This precise control mechanism facilitates fine chewing movements and detection of food texture. When all natural teeth have been lost, this mechanism is also lost and this impacts significantly on chewing performance.

Selection of abutment teeth for overdentures

The principle criteria for selection of teeth as suitable for overdenture abutments are:

* At least two roots should be retained.
* They should be symmetrically distributed.
* It should be possible to create a dome shape with or without restorations.
* At least 50% bone support remains.
* Endodontic procedures should be possible.

For complete overdenture prostheses, at least two roots should be kept for support. These should be symmetrically distributed in the dental arch to ensure stability of the denture. Failure to follow these guidelines is likely to result in a denture that "rocks" as it pivots around a single root surface or roots not symmetrically distributed. The roots chosen for overdenture support should have a reasonable degree of bone support, and as a general rule of thumb there should be at least 50% bone support. A moderate degree of mobility is not a contraindication, as this is likely to diminish once the crown root ratio has been reduced with preparation of the crown of the tooth. It should be possible to create a dome shape either by preparing the roots or by inserting cast dome-shaped restorations into the root canals. Teeth that have decayed below the alveolar crest of bone are not suitable as overdenture abutments. A further relative contraindication would be if the tooth were not suitable for endodontic procedures. This sometimes occurs in older adults where deposition of secondary dentine occludes the root canals and makes access for instrumentation along the whole of the root canal difficult or impossible. In some cases, the clinician may choose to use such roots as long as there is no evidence of apical pathology. A further option is to choose an adjacent root that is more favourable for endodontic procedures.

Endodontic considerations

In most circumstances, root canal therapy is required and this should be undertaken using standard guidelines. A variety of materials can be used to fill access cavities, and the most commonly used are dental amalgam, composite resins and glass ionomer cements. Whichever material is chosen, it is vital that the material is well retained – the clinician should remove 2–3 mm of gutta percha from the root canal to ensure adequate bulk of material is placed in the access cavity. Should the access cavity restoration fall out or fail, there is a distinct possibility of coronal leakage with infection of the root canal system. In some cases, the root canal is very small due to deposition of secondary dentine. In these cases, the clinician has the option of not undertaking endodontic therapy and monitoring the tooth for signs and symptoms of infection.

Abutment tooth preparation

The teeth selected as overdenture abutments should have endodontic therapy prior to tooth preparation. This should be undertaken prior to preparation of the overdenture abutment. Typical preparation features are shown in Fig 10-2. The tooth should be "domed" leaving approximately 3 mm of tooth tissue supra-gingivally. The edges of the preparation should be rounded, and the centre of tooth flattened. It is important not to reduce the abutments to the level of the gingival margin, as this will lead to gingival inflammation when the denture covers the abutments. It is also important not to under prepare abutment teeth, as leaving too much tooth tissue potentially weakens the overdenture (Fig 10-3).

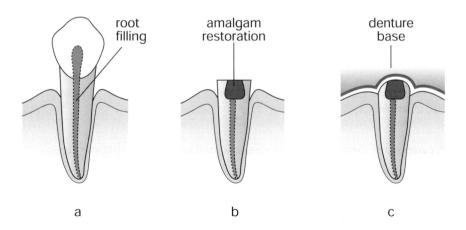

Fig 10-2 Preparation features for an overdenture abutment. Note the dome shape.

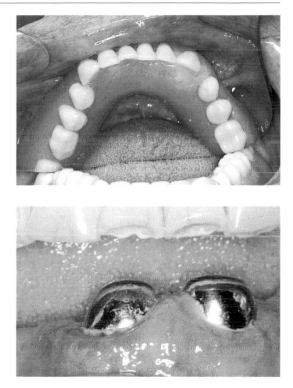

Fig 10-3 Underprepared overdenture abutment (43) This has left little room for acrylic, thus weakening the denture.

Fig 10-4 Cast gold dome copings used to support an overdenture when ideal dome shape cannot be achieved with natural tooth.

When a regular domed tooth preparation is not possible owing to the presence of a previous restoration or caries, a cast gold alloy coping can be used (Fig 10-4). This involves preparing the root canal to retain a post, recording an impression and having a post and dome made in the laboratory. This is cemented into place using a cement system of choice, and the overdenture is then constructed.

Overdenture construction – clinical and laboratory procedures

Complete overdentures can be made by converting existing transitional RPDs or using a replacement technique.

Immediate overdenture procedure

In the immediate overdenture situation, the procedure involves either converting an existing transitional partial denture to a complete overdenture or providing an immediate replacement overdenture. The latter procedure is commonly applicable in tooth wear cases.

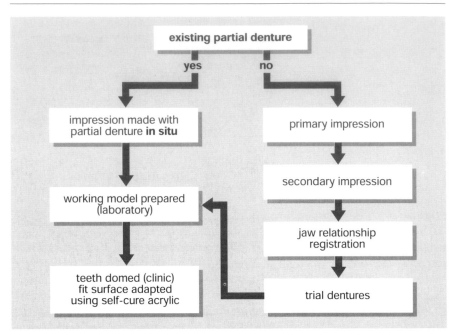

Fig 10-5 Clinical and laboratory stages in the construction of overdentures.

In the case of an older adult, the clinician may have decided that the patient has to go through a transition phase of wearing an RPD prior to a full over-denture. These dentures are normally constructed so than they can be easily converted into a complete overdenture. The rationale for providing such a prosthesis is to aid the patient in adapting to a removable prosthesis. Once the patient has adapted, teeth of a poor prognosis can be extracted in a planned fashion. The clinical and laboratory steps are shown in Fig 10-5.

- An impression is made of the denture in situ using either irreversible hydrocolloid or elastomeric impression material.
- Once the working model is cast, the clinician should trim the teeth that are to be retained as overdenture abutments to the desired shape. Teeth scheduled for extraction are removed from the cast. The denture teeth are then waxed onto the cast and processed into acrylic.
- Once the denture is returned to the clinic, the natural teeth selected as overdenture abutments are prepared to a dome shape and remaining teeth extracted. The processed denture is tried in and adapted to the abutment teeth using self-cured acrylic resin.

In some cases, the patient has not had a transitional partial denture. The

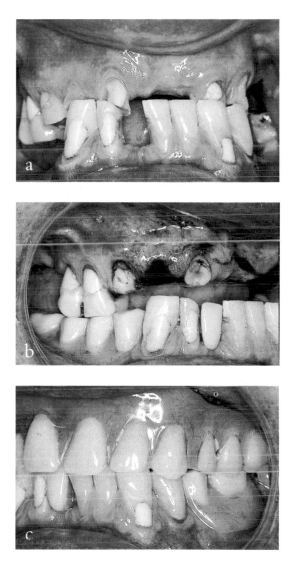

Fig 10-6 Clinical stages in the construction of complete immediate overdenture: (a) initial presentation; (b) extractions and tooth preparation at denture delivery stage; (c) immediate postoperative result.

patient in Fig 10-6a had lost a number of teeth and had become unhappy about the appearance of his teeth and requested treatment to address this. He had not previously worn a partial denture and it was decided to extract some maxillary teeth and retain some as overdenture abutments. Primary

113

and secondary impressions were made using irreversible hydrocolloid. The jaw relationships were registered and a trial denture stage was undertaken to confirm the adequacy of the occlusal relationship. The teeth to be retained as overdenture abutments were then prepared on the working cast. Teeth that were to be extracted were removed from the working cast and the denture processed. Once the denture was returned to the clinic, the abutment teeth were prepared and extractions were undertaken (Fig 10-6b). The denture was modified using self-curing acrylic resin to adapt it to the prepared abutment teeth. The tissues healed uneventfully and the patient adapted well to wearing the denture (Fig 10-6c). After a suitable healing period, a replacement complete overdenture was constructed.

Complete Replacement Overdentures

When replacement of the immediate overdenture is required, the denture is constructed using the same clinical and laboratory stages as for a complete denture.

- Primary impressions are recorded and special trays are constructed.
- When recording final impressions, the clinician should consider the differential support offered by the overdenture abutments and the remainder of the denture bearing area. If no allowance is made for this, then the denture is likely to be unstable in function, as it will tend to pivot around the overdenture abutments. The most effective technique for addressing this problem is to use a selective-pressure impression technique. The instruction for the construction of the special impression tray should specify a close-fitting tray with holes placed in the area corresponding to the abutments. At the next appointment, the tray should be checked, and, if satisfactory, the clinician should record a mucocompressive impression using green stick tracing compound and Zinc Oxide Eugenol impression paste. The material that has flowed through the holes should then be removed and the impression reseated. Finally, impression plaster should be placed through the holes onto the abutment teeth with the base in situ. The final impression should have a recording of the edentate denture-bearing tissues in a compressed state, with a static impression of the abutment teeth. In theory, this should reduce the problems caused by the differential in support offered by the abutment teeth and the edentulous areas.
- Jaw registration, trial dentures and denture delivery stages are then undertaken.

Precision attachment mechanisms

In most cases, the shape of the overdenture abutments, coupled with appropriate use of tissue undercuts, is sufficient to ensure adequate retention of overdentures. In some cases, the clinician has various options for enhancing retention using precision attachments or magnets. Situations where this is likely to arise include:

- Elderly adults provided with a complete denture for the first time.
- Patients likely to have poor muscular control, such as those with Parkinson's disease or post-cerebrovascular accident (stroke).
- Patients with cleft palate or post tumour resection.

The possible attachment mechanisms are:
- bars
- ball attachments/press studs
- magnets.

When contemplating the use of precision attachments, the clinician should be certain that they are necessary and likely to be of benefit to the patient. They are expensive and increase the length of treatment time. They also increase maintenance requirements. Finally, they exert significant stresses on the abutment teeth. There is no evidence to indicate that any of these mechanisms is better than another and the choice is often down to the clinician's preference.

There is some evidence to suggest that magnets exert less force on the peri odontium than precision attachments and therefore are indicated in teeth with reduced periodontal support.

Having selected abutment teeth as previously described, these teeth must have endodontic treatment using conventional endodontic treatment guidelines. The root canal should be prepared for a cast post restoration. As the teeth will not be restored with crowns, it is not necessary to prepare the root canal to within 3 mm of the apex. The attachment component is soldered to a cast diaphragm and the reciprocal component incorporated into the denture. When magnets are used, the copings in the teeth should be made of palladium cobalt alloy. Cobalt samarium magnets are housed in the denture base and a magnetic attraction is created between the copings and the magnets (Fig 10-7).

Maintenance

Despite the many potential benefits of overdentures, there is a major requirement for maintenance. A key element in achieving success with overdentures is that the patient understands the importance of the prevention of

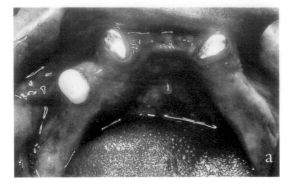

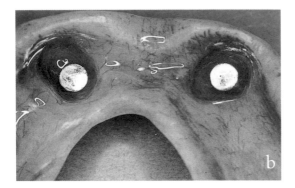

Fig 10-7 Overdenture using magnets for retention: (a) posts and diaphragm in the abutments; (b) magnets in the impression surface of the denture.

oral disease. Coverage of the root faces with the overdenture reduces access of teeth to saliva. This increases the potential for caries and development of gingival inflammation (Fig 10-8). It should also be considered that many patients requiring overdentures might not have satisfactory plaque control procedures. At the outset of treatment to provide overdentures, the patient should be instructed in how to clean plaque from the root faces. This can be done using tufted interdental brushes or electric toothbrushes. Further considerations include:

- The use of fluoride toothpastes.
- The denture should be left out at night time and steeped in a denture cleaner.
- Instruction to use a fluoride mouth rinse daily.
- Professional application of fluoride gels or varnishes.

The patient should have regular reviews with the dentist and the abutments must be checked carefully for signs of caries and/or periodontal disease. These measures will reduce the risk of loss of abutment teeth and consequent eden-

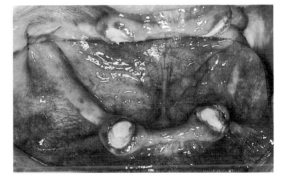

Fig 10-8 Deterioration of abutment teeth due to caries beneath a complete overdenture. These teeth were extracted and a complete replacement denture was provided.

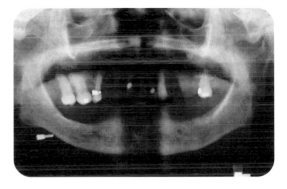

Fig 10-9 Radiograph showing an edentulous mandible opposed by a dentate maxillary arch. The uneven occlusal plane makes it difficult to achieve balanced articulation for the denture, and pain beneath in the lower jaw is common. This situation should be avoided if at all possible.

tulism. Of major relevance is the loss of mandibular teeth when the maxillary arch is dentate (Fig 10-9). This is a very complex clinical situation and achieving balanced articulation of the complete denture and tolerance of occlusal forces is very challenging. Clearly, every effort should be made to avoid this situation.

Implants versus overdentures

With the advent of implants, it could be argued that the indications for use of natural tooth roots to retain and support dentures have decreased. Implant-retained overdentures are not affected by caries or periodontal diseases and of course do not require endodontic therapy. However, surgery is required to place dental implants, and older adults in particular may refuse to have surgery. A further consideration is the cost involved in implant therapy, and this could be beyond the financial resources of older adults. To date, there have not been any studies that directly compare implant-retained overdentures and removable overdentures. It seems logical to suggest that there is a

117

place for both treatment modalities in the management of the older adult, and one should not discount either.

Conclusions

- Retention of some natural teeth to support a complete overdenture offers significant benefit.
- Coupled with these benefits, the clinician should be aware that overdentures are associated with a high burden of maintenance.
- Retention may be enhanced by use of precision attachments, but these also increase cost and maintenance requirements. Consequently, these should be used only when deemed essential.

Further Reading

Basker R, Ralph J, Harrison A, Watson C. Overdentures in General Dental Practice. 3rd ed. London: Macmillan, 1993.

Index

Quintessentials for General Dental Practitioners Series

in 36 volumes

Editor-in-Chief: Professor Nairn H F Wilson

The Quintessentials for General Dental Practitioners Series covers basic principles and key issues in all aspects of modern dental medicine. Each book can be read as a stand-alone volume or in conjunction with other books in the series.

Publication date, approximately

Oral Surgery and Oral Medicine, Editor: John G Meechan

Practical Dental Local Anaesthesia	available
Practical Oral Medicine	Spring 2004
Practical Conscious Sedation	Autumn 2003
Practical Surgical Dentistry	Spring 2004

Imaging, Editor: Keith Horner

Interpreting Dental Radiographs	available
Panoramic Radiology	Autumn 2003
Twenty-first Century Dental Imaging	Autumn 2004

Periodontology, Editor: Iain L C Chapple

Understanding Periodontal Diseases: Assessment and Diagnostic Procedures in Practice	available
Decision-Making for the Periodontal Team	Autumn 2003
Successful Periodontal Therapy – A Non-Surgical Approach	Autumn 2003
Periodontal Management of Children and Adolescents	Autumn 2003
Periodontal Medicine in Practice	Spring 2004

Implantology, Editor: Lloyd J Searson

Implants for the General Practitioner	available
Managing Orofacial Pain in General Dental Practice	Spring 2003

Endodontics, Editor: John M Whitworth

Rational Root Canal Treatment in Practice	available
Managing Endodontic Failure in Practice	Autumn 2003
Managing Dental Trauma in Practice	Autumn 2003
Managing the Vital Pulp in Practice	Autumn 2004

Prosthodontics, Editor: P Finbarr Allen

Teeth for Life for Older Adults	available
Complete Dentures – from Planning to Problem Solving	Autumn 2003
Removable Partial Dentures – A Systematic Approach	Autumn 2003
Fixed Prosthodontics for the General Dental Practitioner	Autumn 2003
Occlusion: A Theoretical and Team Approach	Autumn 2004

Operative Dentistry, Editor: Paul A Brunton

Decision-Making in Operative Dentistry	available
Applied Dental Materials in Operative Dentistry	Spring 2003
Aesthetic Dentistry	Autumn 2003
Successful Indirect Restorations in General Practice	Spring 2004

Paediatric Dentistry/Orthodontics, Editor: Marie Therese Hosey

Child Taming: How to Cope with Children in Dental Practice	Spring 2003
Paediatric Cariology	Autumn 2003
Treatment Planning for the Developing Dentition	Autumn 2003

General Dentistry and Practice Management, Editor: Raj Rattan

The Business of Dentistry	available
Risk Management in General Dental Practice	Spring 2003
Practice Management for the Dental Team	Autumn 2003
Application of Information Technology in General Dental Practice	Spring 2004
Quality Assurance in General Dental Practice	Autumn 2004
Evidence-Based Care in General Dental Practice	Spring 2005

Quintessence Publishing Co. Ltd., London